W0036326

Global Research in Gender, Sexuality and Health

Series Editors
Ellen Annandale
Sociology
University of York Sociology
York, North Yorkshire, UK

Xiaodong Lin
Department of Sociology
University of York Department of Sociology
York, UK

Global Research in Gender, Sexuality and Health brings together original, forward-looking research on gender, sexuality and health at a time of far-reaching and complex global transformations in each of these areas. The associations between these realms are being reconfigured by global social change in different ways and with different consequences for the experience of illness and delivery of healthcare in local and national contexts. New experiences of health and illness are also being driven by the increased global mobility of bodies and illnesses and the growing securitization of illness. In turn, these are challenging conventional ways of thinking about gender, gender, sexualities and the body and call for novel conceptual approaches that are a better fit for an understanding of health in a 'global age'. This interdisciplinary series aims to showcase original research monographs and edited collections of interest to an international readership. Studies from the Global South are particularly encouraged, to help reflect on and revise knowledge of gender, sexuality and health beyond a Eurocentric perspective.

More information about this series at
http://www.palgrave.com/gp/series/15916

Nana K. Poku

Sexual and Reproductive Health and Rights in Sub-Saharan Africa

palgrave
macmillan

Nana K. Poku
University of KwaZulu-Natal
Durban, South Africa

ISSN 2523-7683   ISSN 2523-7691   (electronic)
Global Research in Gender, Sexuality and Health
ISBN 978-981-15-8501-2   ISBN 978-981-15-8502-9   (eBook)
https://doi.org/10.1007/978-981-15-8502-9

© The Editor(s) (if applicable) and The Author(s), under exclusive licence to Springer Nature Singapore Pte Ltd. 2020
This work is subject to copyright. All rights are solely and exclusively licensed by the Publisher, whether the whole or part of the material is concerned, specifically the rights of translation, reprinting, reuse of illustrations, recitation, broadcasting, reproduction on microfilms or in any other physical way, and transmission or information storage and retrieval, electronic adaptation, computer software, or by similar or dissimilar methodology now known or hereafter developed.
The use of general descriptive names, registered names, trademarks, service marks, etc. in this publication does not imply, even in the absence of a specific statement, that such names are exempt from the relevant protective laws and regulations and therefore free for general use.
The publisher, the authors and the editors are safe to assume that the advice and information in this book are believed to be true and accurate at the date of publication. Neither the publisher nor the authors or the editors give a warranty, expressed or implied, with respect to the material contained herein or for any errors or omissions that may have been made. The publisher remains neutral with regard to jurisdictional claims in published maps and institutional affiliations.

Cover pattern © Melisa Hasan

This Palgrave Pivot imprint is published by the registered company Springer Nature Singapore Pte Ltd.
The registered company address is: 152 Beach Road, #21-01/04 Gateway East, Singapore 189721, Singapore

Contents

Acronyms

ACHPR	African Charter on Human and Peoples' Rights
AIDS	Acquired Immune Deficiency Syndrome
ART	Antiretroviral treatment
ARV	Antiretroviral
APRM	African Peer Review Mechanism
AU	African Union
AWP	African Women's Protocol
BRICS	Brazil, Russia, India, China and South Africa
CEDAW	Convention on the Elimination of Discrimination Against Women
DALY	Disability-Adjusted Life Year
DHS	Demographic and Health Surveys
DOTS	Directly Observed Treatment, Short-Course
EAC	East African Community
EAHRC	East African Health Research Commission
ESA	East and Southern African
EU	European Union
GDP	Gross domestic product
HIV	Human immunodeficiency virus
HPV	Human papillomavirus infection
ICCPR	International Covenant on Civil and Political Rights
ICESCR	International Covenant on Economic, Social and Cultural Rights
ICPD	International Conference on Population and Development
IMCI	Integrated Management of Childhood Illness
LGBTQ	Lesbian, gay, bisexual and transgender
LMIC	Low-income and middle-income countries
MDGs	Millennium Development Goals
MICS	Multiple Indicator Cluster Surveys

OECD	Organisation for Economic Co-operation and Development
PEPFAR	The United States President's Emergency Plan for AIDS Relief
PLHIV	People living with HIV
SADC	The Southern African Development Community
SARS	Severe Acute Respiratory Syndrome
SDGs	Sustainable Development Goals
SDH	Social determinants of health
SRH	Sexual and reproductive health
SRHR	Sexual and reproductive health rights
SSA	Sub-Saharan Africa
STD	Sexually transmitted disease
STI	Sexually transmitted infection
TB	Tuberculosis
UHC	Universal Health Coverage
UN	United Nations
UNAIDS	Joint United Nations Programme on HIV and AIDS
UNFPA	United Nations Population Fund
UNICEF	United Nations Children's Fund
USD	United States Dollars
WHO	World Health Organization

LIST OF TABLES

CHAPTER 1

Introduction

Sexual and Reproductive Health and the Human Condition

Abstract The Introduction is a thematic overview of the book, offering a rationale for why the focus is on a rights-based approach to sexual and reproductive health in sub-Saharan Africa.

Keywords Human nature • Disease • Rights • Sub-Saharan Africa

Properly speaking, nothing is true about human nature that is not true of every one of us—hence the difficulty of creating a definition that is at once both sufficiently encompassing but also precise. Despite our knowledge of human physiology and cognition, the scholarly insights from philosophy, psychology, social psychology, sociology and anthropology and from our lived experience, the search for an indisputably true 'human nature' is an endlessly elusive quest. Much the same applies to many of the larger configurations of the human condition because verifiable facts are conditioned by, and interact with, the irreducible dynamism and complexity of natural and human systems.

It is through the conjunction of biological processes and human behaviours that much of the worst and most widespread forms of human disease and other forms of ill health are facilitated and embedded. This is not to discount the role of pathogens, but a recognition that people are not mere

© The Author(s), under exclusive license to Springer Nature Singapore Pte Ltd. 2020
N. K. Poku, *Sexual and Reproductive Health and Rights in Sub-Saharan Africa*, Global Research in Gender, Sexuality and Health, https://doi.org/10.1007/978-981-15-8502-9_1

bodies in space. Contexts matter for the full range of human harms and debility. We might usefully paraphrase Randolph Kent's insight into natural disasters, substituting 'disease' for 'disaster' '[Diseases] are the consequence of the way humanity lives its "normal life". [Disease] agents do not foster vulnerability, but the ways in which human beings organise their social and economic lives do.'[1] One need not look far for what Paul Farmer has termed 'biological expressions of social inequality'[2]—tuberculosis being an obvious and persistent case in point. And from the start of the Covid-19 pandemic, it was clear that the rates of infection and mortality in US cities are disproportionately high in African-American neighbourhoods.[3]

Susceptibility to both infectious and non-infectious disease as well as the prospects for good health generally can be magnified or diminished by what are commonly termed the social determinants of health.[4] Many of these are readily identifiable because they are structural, combining numerous and often varied elements to form complex conditions not amenable to linear 'solutions.' These include poverty, poor housing, low educational attainment and unemployment. The pervasiveness and inertia of these and other socio-economic and socio-political fixtures also shape the more dynamic, self-determining elements of human health—a point implicit in health-related legislation intended to bring about a re-orientation of individual behaviours that are deleterious to health.

But the boundaries between structural and behavioural factors in shaping health outcomes for individuals and societies are not entirely distinct; societies are not homogeneous and cultural norms are not monolithic; and individual deliberation is not detached from circumstantial influences—in the worst cases, like unaffordable or inaccessible health care, 'choice' is highly constrained by social determinants. Writ large, sexual and reproductive health offers countless intersections between the many realms that comprise the human condition. These are typically clustered together in ever-shifting patterns to provide the foundation for the richness of life, with all its pleasures and perils, sources of meaning and menace, and its biological and personal imperatives, including the procreative urge. The intensely personal and deeply meaningful aspects of sexuality and reproduction find expression in social contexts, not only in tensioned relationships between the personal and the political, or individual values and cultural norms but also at larger scales, including the political economy of health at national and international levels.[5] Government injunctions in the form of incentives and disincentives meant to increase or diminish national birth rates[6] are an example of the ways in which the phrase, 'the personal is political' finds particularly striking expression.

Although statistical indicators for the purpose of framing public health policy are not always readily available or completely reliable,[7] at the largest scales, they are vital for epidemiological purposes and at least broadly indicative of health conditions for which causal elements are difficult to discern and untangle. So it is that we know how people become infected by human immunodeficiency virus (HIV), but comprehending how adolescents in high-prevalence countries calculate risk requires careful, on-the-ground behavioural research; likewise, why in some countries where abortion is legal, the number of unsafe abortions remains alarmingly high.

What makes the many issues, conditions and dynamics comprising sexual and reproductive health (SRH) so compelling is their vital importance for both individual well-being and public health at every scale, together with their universality—that is, a fundamental part of our shared humanity; and what makes SRH so intellectually and practically difficult is that the clear health outcomes—ranging from fertility rates to deaths from Acquired Immune Deficiency Syndrome (AIDS)—emerge from numerous other conditions and calculations, ranging from international organization and the culturally conditioned meanings of gender to our most private and intimate life choices. We conceptualize sexual health and reproductive health jointly even though for certain conditions or outcomes there is not always a direct causal link between the two distinct realms—but in the course of ordinary human flourishing, the two routinely defy abstraction from one another. The larger conception also restores us to the unity of life and to an outline appreciation of why the sources of so many individual debilities cannot be addressed as clinical matters alone.

In addition, conceptualizing sexual and reproductive health jointly has for decades been fundamental to comprehending and addressing the HIV/AIDS pandemic; and for placing individual issues within contexts which prompt the investigation of correlations for causal relations—not least poverty and gender-based discrimination, which imparted much to the substance and orientation of the Millennium Development Goals (2000–15). In short, any serious consideration of SRH beyond statistics—and certainly for the purposes of human betterment—obliges us to engage with the many non-medical realms that shape our lives—the cultural, legal, political and economic structures through which public health is organized.

These matters are inescapably political because they deal with power, responsibility and accountability. The expectation that the social contract between citizens and their states should now include at least some basic provision for public health and the alleviation of preventable suffering has been a key feature of the gradual development of democratic politics.[8] Contestation about what such measures should comprise, and how they should be paid for, continues, most notably around a growing normative expectation of Universal Health Coverage, not confined to the most resource-constrained states. At the same time, laws that seek to regulate or prohibit behaviours at the heart of human sexuality (expressions of gender identity; same-sex relationships; transactional sex; contraception; abortion) are often lodged within a matrix of not always homogenous cultural norms, religious beliefs and strained personal circumstances. These and related issues are often played out against and interwoven with rights claims.

We can distinguish rights as citizen entitlements (typically, national constitutional provisions) and human rights—universal and inalienable. All rights contestations have deep roots, in line with the broader and continuing adjustments between states and citizens, responsibilities and rights. The disappointments occasioned by our failures to enact positive human rights include the sensitivities of many states—hence the foreshortening of SRH rights in Sustainable Development Goal 5.6 to 'ensure universal access to sexual and reproductive health and reproductive rights.' It is precisely because sexual and reproductive health is fundamental of the human condition that they engender so many moral sensitivities, taboos and anxieties; and for the same reason, they are also at the heart of the human rights regime. Our disappointments should be tempered by recognition of the normative power of rights standards and demands on individual states and the international system and in the lived expectations of so many people. The tensions and struggles between universalist ideals on one hand and socio-political and socio-cultural values and interests on the other will persist, played out in the lives of individuals and families no less than in halls of government. But these are not essentially philosophical debates: throughout the world, the impacts of the AIDS pandemic have been a powerful solvent on resistances to a more open and forthright acknowledgement and acceptance of the realities of human sexuality and has brought many hitherto side-lined SRH issues (gender inequalities; marginalized/criminalized populations with multiple health vulnerabilities; inequitable and/or unaffordable SRH services) to the fore.

The subject of this book is sexual and reproductive health *rights*, with sub-Saharan Africa (SSA) as the regional focus. In aggregate statistical terms, the region suffers from seriously entrenched and challenging SRH issues, but with large and noteworthy state and sub-state variations in the operative cultural, social and economic drivers; and also in terms of individual states' capacity to engage with them on a sustainable basis, particularly in a climate of overseas development assistance retrenchment. Far from sub-Saharan Africa being a region either uniformly burdened or lacking in key capacities, its uniqueness for the purposes of a study on sexual and reproductive health rights is the variety of the nations that comprise it and their efforts over many years to engage African regional and continental organizations in developing responses to SRH issues, both within the region and in conjunction with the broader worldwide responses to advance SRH.

There is little in the experience of SSA societies or their governments that is unique except in terms of degree and in the legacies of their histories and the cultural particulars that shape the sexual and reproductive health of its peoples. For all that the social determinants of sexual and reproductive health vary across the world, we share a common humanity, more obviously visible in human sexuality and human continuance than in any other human particular. That they also entail so much preventable ill health and suffering is a rationale for engagement that should include us all.

NOTES

1. Randolph C. Kent, *Anatomy of Disaster Relief: The International Network in Action* (London: Pinter Publishers, 1987), p. 4.
2. Paul Framer, *Infections and Inequalities: The Modern Plagues* (Berkeley: University of California Press, 1999).
3. In Chicago, black Americans account for 68 per cent of the city's 118 deaths and 52 per cent of the roughly 5000 confirmed coronavirus cases, despite making up just 30 per cent of the city's population. That means they are dying at a rate nearly six times higher than that of white Chicagoans—a striking disparity that is also starting to emerge in other major cities. Meagan Flynn, '"Those numbers take your breath away": Covid-19 is hitting Chicago's black neighbourhoods much harder than others, officials say,' *Washington Post*, 7 April 2020.
4. Michael Marmot and Richard G. Wilkinson (eds), *Social Determinants of Health* (Oxford: Oxford University Press, 2005).

5. Maria Tanyag, 'Depleting fragile bodies: the political economy of sexual and reproductive health in crisis situations,' *Review of International Studies*, Vol. 44, part 4 (2018), pp. 654–71; Peter Kelly and Jo Pike (eds), *Neo-Liberalism and austerity: the moral economies of young people's health and well-being* (London: Palgrave Macmillan, 2017).

6. David Howden and Yang Zhou, 'China's One-Child Policy: Some Unintended Consequences,' *Economic Affairs,* 17 October 2014, https://doi-org.ezp.lib.cam.ac.uk/10.1111/ecaf.12098; Suzanne Bonner Dipanwita Sarkar, 'Who responds to fertility-boosting incentives? Evidence from pro-natal policies in Australia,' *Demographic Research*, Vol. 42, article 18 (13 March 2020), pp. 513–48.

7. Carla AbouZahr and Ties Boerma, 'Health information systems: the foundations of public health,' *Bulletin of the World Health Organization* 83, 8 (August 2005), pp. 578–83.

8. Nana Poku and Jesper Sunderwall, **'Political responsibility and global health,'** *Third World Quarterly* 39(3), pp. 471–86.

CHAPTER 2

The Principle of Sexual and Reproductive Health and Why It Is Central to Broad Advancements in Human Health and Development in Sub-Saharan Africa

Abstract This chapter begins with a consideration of the strongly relational character of human health by outlining the centrality of gender. The following sub-sections present conceptual understandings of both sexual and reproductive health, followed by definitions of the terms that enjoy a broad consensus. The first section ends with a consideration of sexual and reproductive health as a configuration of closely inter-related issues—including but not limited to HIV and AIDS. The second half of the chapter offers a rationale for the sub-Saharan focus of the study and introduces political, normative and socio-legal perspectives that will inform subsequent chapters.

Keywords Sexual • Reproductive • Gender • HIV
• Sub-Saharan Africa

Gender and Health

The incidence and patterns of human disease cannot be reduced to bacterial and viral dynamics, or to the presence of vectors that carry them such as mosquitoes and ticks. And although there are place-specific variables

© The Author(s), under exclusive license to Springer Nature Singapore Pte Ltd. 2020
N. K. Poku, *Sexual and Reproductive Health and Rights in Sub-Saharan Africa*, Global Research in Gender, Sexuality and Health, https://doi.org/10.1007/978-981-15-8502-9_2

which heighten risk (for instance, those diseases specific to the tropics), the largest part of human disease vulnerability is relational—that is, the structural, social and interpersonal bases of social organization and individual behaviours. So for example, the steep rise in the incidence and prevalence of tuberculosis from the eighteenth century is closely correlated with the rise of industrialization and urbanization. Similarly, there is nothing 'natural' about inequality and poverty, discrimination and malnourishment, all of which markedly increase susceptibility to a variety of diseases and forms of debilitation.[1]

Socialization is a sine qua non for the full development of personhood. This not only entails primary forms of human bonding and the acquisition of language but also rules and prohibitions; forms of authority and sanctions, the bases of cooperation and competition; the division of labour. Many of the norms which give societies their coherence and stability embed hierarchies of power—and some of the most important of these are explicitly gendered, nowhere more visibly than in matters pertaining to the construction of personal identity, the conduct of sexual relations, procreation and the composition of families. Differences in customs and taboos, and allowances for individuals vary considerably across and even within cultures, but female sexuality is monitored everywhere; and the expectations around women acquiring professional expertise and financial independence and forms and degrees of equality remain quite repressive in many parts of the world. The male prerogative, exercised through laws, customs or by structural means (self-policing families and communities; the burden of time-consuming physical labour; few if any worthwhile opportunities for paid employment) is still very much intact. And perhaps the best means open to women—and especially poor ones—of creating and expanding a compass of personal autonomy is through controlling their fertility. But women's control of their fertility is often sited within marriages or partnerships that preclude either meaningful choice or negotiation.

Highly gendered and unequal power/authority dynamics in sexual and familial relationships are reinforced in many cases by the culturally embedded expectations of women themselves, the absence of practical means for them to live independently or assertively and fear of being ostracized. At the same time, culturally sanctioned sex and gender roles are no more likely to be self-serving (for men), inconsistent or hypocritical than any other cultural artefact. These are, after all, relations of power—and they can manifest in a variety of ways: what counts as 'promiscuity' and how it is perceived socially; a casual approach to birth control (and/or the man's refusal to sanction it), a disregard for safe sex; coerced or transactional sex; very early female sexual debut; and ensuring paternity through female genital mutilation. Many of these kinds of behaviours, to varying degrees socially endorsed, or at least unsanctioned, greatly increase vulnerability to sexually transmitted diseases—for men as well as for women—as well as a much wider range of outcomes, unwanted pregnancies not least. Both formal and informal proscriptions against homosexuality and non-traditional gender identities are also key manifestations of the ways in which gender—and by extension, sexual behaviours—are structured for purposes that do not accommodate the variety of ways of being human.

But the gender and sexual politics of everyday life also have wider, encompassing contexts which shape and influence them, most importantly the socio-economic conditions to which societies adjust, especially since there are now few if any that are not subject to the rapidly shifting currents of globalization. Gender and gendered politics feature at every scale of the organization of political community, including the largest: global restructuring, migration, the political economy of human trafficking and sex work, 'development' in its many meanings and war and violence, to name but a few.[2]

It is impossible to imagine that a country in which the majority (or even a sizeable proportion) live in poverty could have positive, aggregate health statistics in any significant particular. And although the more pernicious forms of gender politics can be generated, shaped and even reinforced by life in slums and conflict zones, the absence of clean water and sanitation, poisoned or degraded land, unsafe working conditions and an inability to secure monetized commodities, gender and gender relations are not at the root of the appalling and preventable human suffering that stem from indecent living conditions.

Yet one need not focus solely on sites of poverty and degradation to record high and largely preventable incidences of morbidity and mortality arising from the fundamentals of human coexistence and continuance, particularly with respect to sexual and reproductive health.[3] And as we have reviewed here briefly, the values, beliefs and circumstances that combine to facilitate these outcomes are highly gendered.

CONCEPTUALIZING SEXUAL AND REPRODUCTIVE HEALTH

For a range of practical purposes, the concepts 'sexual health' and 'reproductive health' are necessary abstractions not only from the bodily integrity of human health in its fullest sense, but also from their cognitive, psychological, behavioural and relational aspects; and from their socio-cultural and socio-political contexts. The interests and values that drive constructions of gender and identity are fully operative in matters sexual and reproductive; and sexual and reproductive health is similarly constructed: they are neither entirely objective nor comprehensive. Both terms carry a risk of distortion and a counter-productive narrowing of focus, since how we conceive and construct these and other aspects of human health has a powerful bearing on the orientation and priorities of public health and public health promotion. For example, with respect to sexual health,

> there is a tacit assumption that sexual health is solely concerned with the individual's avoidance of infection. In the case of HIV, this has resulted in health promotion efforts almost exclusively concerned to protect the uninfected rather than addressing the sexual needs of people already infected. The cultural and political climate of the recent past can also help to explain the prevalence of an individualism which, against common sense ('it takes two to tango'), epidemiology and personal experience, sought to explain complex, dyadic, potentially pleasurable social behaviour solely in terms of individuals' disease-avoiding cognitions.[4]

In much the same way, the usefulness of abstracting the reproductive health of women as a means of addressing serious public health deficiencies has entailed a refinement of reproductive health to a focus on pregnancy and childbirth which was 'appropriate historically [because] in low-income and middle-income countries (LMICs), the improvements in maternal deaths around childbirth were very modest during most of the twentieth century, prompting a maternal and child health approach as a worldwide campaign to improve maternal health.'[5] However, the prioritization, utility and urgency of these abstractions ('reproductive health' and 'maternal health') are subject to contexts which extend beyond an unchanging human physiology to embrace the broader dynamics shaping human health—and these too are subject to change:

> In view of the remarkable transitions in the health needs and roles of women, a narrow conception of maternal health undervalues the burden of illness faced by women, because most women live past the age of child bearing. Narrow interpretations of maternal health adversely affect global health priorities, and can lead to a restrictive vision of the needs of women across their

life cycle and restrict their potential to contribute to their families, communities, health systems, societies, and economies.[6]

None of this calls into question the necessity of abstractions for nearly every form of detailed intellectual enquiry or for the crafting and implementation of public policy to address one or another social ill. But as a concept, sexual and reproductive health is concerned with human persons, not portions of anatomy or sites of potential infection. The highly relational nature of sexual and reproductive health, at once intensely personal and socially significant, means that the terms carry a variety of meanings in both the medical and social sciences[7]; nevertheless, broad consensus has been secured around the following and similarly comprehensive definitions:

> Reproductive health is a state of complete physical, mental and social well-being and not merely the absence of disease or infirmity, in all matters relating to the reproductive system and to its functions and processes. Reproductive health therefore implies that people are able to have a satisfying and safe sex life and that they have the capability to reproduce and the freedom to decide if, when and how often to do so. Implicit in this last condition are the right of men and women to be informed and to have access to safe, effective, affordable and acceptable methods of family planning of their choice, as well as other methods of their choice for regulation of fertility which are not against the law, and the right of access to appropriate health-care services that will enable women to go safely through pregnancy and childbirth and provide couples with the best chance of having a healthy infant.[8]

And the World Health Organization (WHO) definition of sexual health has few significant differences with other high-profile characterizations of the term[9]:

> Sexual health is a state of physical, emotional, mental and social well-being related to sexuality; it is not merely the absence of disease, dysfunction or infirmity. Sexual health requires a positive and respectful approach to sexuality and sexual relationships, as well as the possibility of having pleasurable and safe sexual experiences, free of coercion, discrimination and violence. For sexual health to be attained and maintained, the sexual rights of all persons must be respected, protected and fulfilled.[10]

What immediately becomes clear on a reading of these and similar definitions is that although there are many practical reasons for differentiating sexual and reproductive health, they are inextricable—even at the interpersonal level, let alone from a societal/public health perspective, reproductive health depends to varying degrees on a modicum of sexual health. Furthermore, the boundaries between the two are more porous than definitional precision might suggest, as the risk of mother-to-child transmission of HIV makes plain.

Second, any discussion of the attainment of sexual and reproductive health, particularly when considered as having significant impacts on public health or on prevailing social norms, cannot advance very far without engaging a discussion of rights—and in modern states, rights are circumscribed and specified by laws.

Laws governing both sexual conduct and all matters pertaining to procreation as they relate to desired social orders differ significantly across cultures, but they have ancient historical antecedents[11]; and the taboos that so often inform them are more deeply rooted and more formative of contemporary socio-cultural norms than is commonly acknowledged.[12] In our own time, the enduring and essentially unresolvable tensions between personal liberty and restrictive law and between private life and public interest find particularly vivid expression in all matters sexual and reproductive; and social norms, particularly when they are legally codified, powerfully reinforce standards and marshal conformity, even in the absence of practical mechanisms for legal enforcement. Laws serve to enshrine certain rights and erect barriers against the assertion and enactment of others. In the sexual and reproductive realms, some are entirely non-controversial (the protection of children and the mentally disabled from exploitation, for example); others pit gender and sexual non-conformity against prohibitive law—homosexuality as a crime, most notably, which does nothing to alter sexual orientation and little to alter behaviour beyond creating hiding/hidden populations, with clear impacts not only for those communities but also for public health more generally.

But many of the laws pertaining to sexual and reproductive health are enabling rather than restrictive: they encode rights (at least at the level of citizen entitlement) to certain freedoms and to pertinent health services, in the interests of both individuals and the public at large. This disposition of states also has a long history, as part of the broader struggles of peoples to oblige their governments to accept a widening span of responsibilities and to hold them to account.[13] Whether and to what degree specific health rights are legally enacted, practically enabled, the resources equitably distributed and/or secured, adequately costed and funded and effectively monitored are matters that site the idea and ideal of health rights within the complexities of human coexistence. 'How shall we live?' is a perennial, the many, often conflicting variables—personal, interpersonal and social— never finally reconciled, but there remains sufficient common interest in maintaining the security and stability of our social orders to make sexual and reproductive health rights and the larger panoply of health regulations a fixture of all contemporary states. The international and national legal provisions for health rights (and for sexual and reproductive rights in particular) will be discussed in Chap. 3.

DELINEATION OF SEXUAL AND REPRODUCTIVE HEALTH ISSUES

Not all sexual and reproductive health (SRH) interventions are medical: they are variously physical and relational; preventive, curative and developmental; and educational. The delineation of topics and issues pertaining to SRH does not automatically encompass either rights or the necessary practical means of securing them, such as fully functional, accessible and affordable health systems. There are also many non-health variables that have a bearing on sexual and reproductive health, such as the availability of clean water and sanitation, the quality of nutrition and the ability of individuals and families to meet out-of-pocket health expenditures. But even at one remove from the environmental, lego-political and financial conditions that make them realizable, the particulars of sexual and reproductive health are considerable in number, closely inter-linked, utterly fundamental to human well-being and are not covered by any single professional or disciplinary approach.

The largest issue looming over sexual and reproductive health for the last three decades has been HIV and AIDS, which manifests in both realms. The yearly costs of HIV prevention and treating people with AIDS have been staggeringly high (currently US$19.1 billion for the AIDS response in low- and middle-income countries, which Joint United Nations Programme on HIV and AIDS (UNAIDS) estimates will stand at 26 billion in 2020 before declining marginally to 23.9 billion by 2030). These costs are set to remain high as a part-consequence of the success of generic antiretroviral (ARV) medicines that transformed AIDS from a life-threatening to a chronic condition. As a result, the 20 million people currently receiving ART will need to remain on a succession of second, third and later generations of drugs for decades to come, as each drug formulation loses its efficacy. Another reason why the financial burden is and will remain very considerable is that despite the achievement of steep reductions in new HIV infections, they remain worryingly high (1.8 million in 2017)—a serious impediment to the best estimates that with sufficient increases in funding, the AIDS epidemic can be ended as a global public health threat by 2030.[14]

National, regional and local responses to HIV and AIDS have necessitated a rapid scaling up of many aspects of health service provision for SRH, since preventive as well as medical responses are the front line in combatting the epidemic. This has included awareness and anti-stigma campaigns, targeted sex education and safe sex programmes, testing, identifying and reaching 'key populations' (sex workers; men who have sex with men; injecting drug users), encouraging male circumcision and the use of condoms; resources devoted to preventing mother-to-child HIV transmission; and, as the rollout of affordable ARVs commenced, administering the drugs and monitoring adherence. The devastating consequences of the epidemic and the range of means necessary to deal with them have revealed how extensive and pervasive are sexual and reproductive dynamics[15] and how they impact every level of human interaction up to and including the global. At the same time, the multidimensional impacts of non-HIV/AIDS SRH failures extend in all directions. For example, 'The maternal health consequences of violence for women are wide-ranging and include fetal loss, low birth weight babies, likelihood of abortion, HIV infection, adolescent pregnancy, unintended pregnancy in general, miscarriage, stillbirth, intrauterine haemorrhage, nutritional deficiency, abdominal pain and other gastrointestinal problems, neurological disorders, chronic pain, disability, clinical depression, anxiety and post-traumatic stress, musculoskeletal injuries and genital injuries.'[16]

So there is vastly more to HIV and AIDS than 'disease' suggests; and there is more to sexual and reproductive health than the more obvious, medically significant outcomes of sex and reproduction. For example, family planning entails a range of sexual and reproductive health issues including safe sex, contraception, maternal health and safe/unsafe abortions, as well as whether the pertinent health service provisions (such as antenatal and neonatal care and midwifery) are accessible and affordable. More profoundly, 'A maternal death […] is as much an outcome of poverty, rights violations, poor access, poor human resources for health and non-existent transport infrastructure as it is an outcome of postpartum haemorrhage or eclampsia. An exclusive focus on clinical interventions, critical though these are, would certainly reduce deaths from cases that report successfully to the health services, but will do very little to prevent those cases that never reached the health services. It has been much easier, therefore to concentrate resources on the concrete interventions that have a tangible and short-term impact than to invest in the translation and operationalisation of complex social phenomena such as changes in societal attitudes, values and protection of human rights.'[17]

In addition, the health impacts of unattended or comprised sexual and reproductive health needs are often multiple; and when not terminal, they frequently cause permanent damage and/or debility:

Every year, an estimated 210 million women have life-threatening complications of pregnancy, often leading to serious disability, and a further half a million women die in pregnancy, childbirth, and the puerperium (more than 99 per cent of these deaths are in developing countries). Three million babies die in the first week of life and about 3·3 million infants are stillborn every year. More than 120 million couples have an unmet need for contraception and 80 million women each year have unwanted or unintended pregnancies, 45 million of which are terminated. Of these 45 million abortions, 19 million are unsafe, 40 per cent of them are done on women aged under 25, and about 68,000 women die every year from complications of unsafe abortion.

An estimated 340 million new cases of four common sexually transmitted bacterial and protozoal infections are acquired every year, at least a third of which affect people aged under 25. Such infections contribute to the global problem of infertility, which affects more than 180 million couples in developing countries (excluding China). [In 2006] Nearly 5 million new HIV infections [in 2006] and 257,000 deaths from cervical cancer every year complete this long and dismal record of sexual and reproductive ill-health. Physical and sexual violence, reported by between one in two and one in six women, is an underlying risk factor for many of these sexual and reproductive health problems.[18]

Table 2.1 illustrates the cross-cutting character of nearly every subject or issue that comes under the heading 'sexual and reproductive health.' While it is by no means exhaustive, it makes clear that in practical terms, the individual and social aspects of these issues arise together, which helps

Table 2.1 The cross-cutting character of factors pertinent to the achievement of sexual and reproductive health

Realm	Issue
Physiological/medical	HIV prevention
Relational	HIV testing and treatment
Behavioural	Other STDs
Educational	Family planning
	Safe sex
Action	Contraception
Prevention	Unwanted pregnancies
Treatment and care	Safe/unsafe abortion
support	
Cure	Antenatal, neonatal and maternal health
Advocacy/anti-stigma/	Partner violence
training	
Conditioning and	**Kinds and degrees of vulnerability**
determining factors	
Social norms	Persecuted sexual/gender identities
Laws/public health policy	Injecting drug users; men who have sex with men; sex workers; prisoners
Health service	Adolescents; disabled; migrants and displaced people; the
infrastructure; access and	poor; individuals without access to health services
affordability	
Poverty; inequality	

to explain their common, underlying sources, the reasons why they are so difficult to deal with in both a systematic and comprehensive manner, the nature of resistance to progressive initiatives, and the difficulties of determining public health priorities for SRH.

This is not to suggest that improvements in SRH are necessarily incidental, patchy or only minutely incremental, or that they can come about only in the most direct, targeted ways. The aggregate statistics from the Millennium Development Goals (MDGs) (2000–15) offer some evidence to the contrary. Although the MDGs omitted a specific goal for SRH, three of the eight MDGs were directly or indirectly concerned with SRH (reduce child mortality; improve maternal health; combat HIV/AIDS, malaria and other diseases); and a further two were dedicated to gender— one directly (promote gender equality and empower women) and one indirectly (achieve universal primary education). A specific commitment to SRH would very likely have facilitated a higher level of achievement of the SRH-related goals; and although not all of the positive MDG outcome data can be ascribed to a concerted effort begun in 2000 (with indirect benefits also arising from the effects of larger development initiatives[19]), the overall results are still positive, with some evidence that international consensus and sustained momentum around a limited and clearly articulated set of development goals and targets can be very effective.[20]

HIV and AIDS have had a profound effect on elevating the profile of sexual and reproductive rights. The initiatives that have provided 20 million people with treatment for AIDS are in part enabled by the large and rapid scale-up of SRH services for both diagnostic and preventive purposes.[21] But stemming the tide of the pandemic has not only overshadowed an appreciation of other advances in SRH (such as the world level of maternal mortality having declined by 45 per cent), but in some places, especially high-incidence/low-income countries, SRH services have become closely tied to policies, infrastructure and programmes that are HIV and AIDS-specific. The outcomes are not always uniformly beneficial. For example, the impetus to integrate family planning and HIV/AIDS services[22] in order to tackle mother-to-child transmission of HIV can have impacts on other aspects of contraception and reproductive health as well as sexual health more generally, especially for those who fear social stigma. Integration of SRH and HIV/AIDS services for purposes of efficiency and cost-saving can have similar impacts.[23]

Aggregate statistics are a key means for international organizations such as the World Health Organization and donor governments to adjust their SRH priorities and to monitor the progress of global health. But the nature, frequency and complexity of sexual and reproductive health issues are determined 'on the ground,' embedded in ways of life which are not amenable to a fixed understanding of the variables or uniform approaches to interventions and/or support. Throughout the world, every expression of human sexuality takes place in contexts that shape its social meanings and to varying degrees the chances of unwanted or harmful outcomes. Individuals engaged in sexual acts and choices need not flaunt predominant norms or prevailing laws for this to be the case, but it is as much the extent of non-conformity and the perception of threat as the incidence of disease and life-threatening conditions that shape sexual and reproductive health as 'issues.' The fear and stigma that attached to HIV and AIDS, particularly as it grew to become a pandemic but persisting even today,[24] demonstrates this. And it is against this background that the assertion of sexual and reproductive health *rights* is so contentious in many parts of the world.

The second half of this chapter will introduce the geographic focus of this study, sub-Saharan Africa (SSA), chosen for three reasons. First, nearly every important aspect of sexual and reproductive health intersects HIV and AIDS—a fact which multiplies, complicates and makes more urgent the challenges of SRH. Sub-Saharan Africa not only has a disproportionate share of the world's HIV-positive people; the socio-legal, political and cultural variety of the states which comprise the region present abundant configurations of SRH/HIV and AIDS challenges, which aggregate statistics cannot capture. Second, despite remarkable advancements in many SSA countries, poverty with all its attendant ills impacts on the fundamentals of health, not least health services infrastructure, access and affordability. The deleterious effects of poverty on sexual and reproductive health are sufficient in number and seriousness to fairly be characterized as 'social determinants.'[25] Third, the demography of Africa critically shapes the prospects for promoting and securing a healthy future for its peoples, because Africa has a very young age profile, with about two-fifths of its population in the 0–14 age bracket and nearly one-fifth (19 per cent) in the 15–24 age bracket. This means that the current 'demographic bulge' of sexually active young adults will grow still further and persist for decades as the generation of 0–14-year-olds also becomes sexually active.

SEXUAL AND REPRODUCTIVE HEALTH IN SUB-SAHARAN AFRICA

As with all other forms of data, aggregate SRH statistics for sub-Saharan Africa are indicative of the extent of issues, but shorn of their political, legal, financial and social contexts, they tell us nothing of causal factors, large differences in key indicators between states, about the capacities of states and communities to make and sustain improvements, or the factors that might best enable them. This is a necessary caveat because 'Africa the country' caricatures persist, while at the same time, economic and financial indicators (Middle Income Country status especially[26]) can mask not only the distribution of poverty internationally[27] but also the extent and levels of inequality within states (and hence the adequacy and affordability of health care). Much the same has been observed about fertility rates in SSA:

The fertility transition has [...] been slow. Fertility in Sub-Saharan Africa has declined, from 6.5 children per woman in 1950–55 to 5.4 in 2005–10, but much less than in other regions. In East Asia, fertility declined from 5.6 to 1.6 over the same period. Once again, regional averages mask large variations—for example, in the Democratic Republic of Congo and Niger, total fertility rates are rising.[28]

Still other key SRH indicators run contrary to negative expectations, such as that in Africa as a whole (albeit with serious anomalies[29]), the neonatal mortality rate per 1000 live birth dropped more than 50 per cent between 1996 and 2016, from 43.6 to 27.2, placing it fractionally ahead of the eastern Mediterranean region.[30] Similarly, the estimated antiretroviral coverage among people living with HIV (as at 2016) included Botswana (83 per cent), Rwanda (80 per cent), Swaziland (79 per cent), Zimbabwe (75 per cent) and Uganda (67 per cent).[31] At the same time, percentage population figures for HIV infection range widely across SSA, with at least five countries that have rates below 3 per cent (Rwanda, Republic of Congo, South Sudan, Chad and Angola), while the worst, Swaziland, stands at 27 per cent, followed by Botswana (25 per cent), Lesotho (23 per cent) and South Africa (18 per cent).

These and other country differentials and anomalies as well as statistical averages in SRH have formative contexts, key actors and complex dynamics.[32] In short, on its own, data have little explanatory power. After all, the root of the AIDS pandemic is relational; and although statistical epidemiology and modelling are vital in tracking and predicting the spread of the disease, both prevention and treatment require a tailoring of programmes to the variety of ways that people contract sexual relations and the knowledge beliefs, dispositions, values and circumstances upon which they act— and again, although there have been some notable improvements in key gender equality indicators in SSA,[33] these are markedly uneven; and gender/gender relations remain fundamental to the spread and distribution of HIV:

> Globally, men and women make up an equal share of the people living with HIV. However, in sub-Saharan Africa, women account for 58 per cent of people living with the virus. For social and physiological reasons, adolescent girls and young women are particularly vulnerable, with HIV infection rates more than double those of males of the same age group.[34]

And throughout much of SSA, the decades-long ravages of the AIDS pandemic have not only placed sexual and reproductive health at the forefront of public health—the two have become all but inextricable:

> HIV is the leading cause of death among women of reproductive age, and it contributes significantly to maternal mortality due both to progression of the disease itself and through higher rates of sepsis, anaemia and other pregnancy-related conditions. Women's and girls' vulnerability to HIV is driven also by gender inequality, including gender-based violence which limits their ability to make safe choices about their sexual and reproductive health.[35]

Indeed, there are few large-scale public health or developmental matters in the region that can be regarded as entirely freestanding from HIV and AIDS. It has long been recognized that the direct and indirect impacts of the AIDS pandemic are not only a public health crisis but also a development issue. Markus Haacker has summarized the national-level financial impacts as follows:

- HIV/AIDS affects material living standards, as measured by GDP and GDP per capita, most directly as a consequence of increased mortality (causing economic disruptions and resulting in a diminished population size), and as private and public HIV/AIDS spending results in diminished investment.
- [However], If the impacts of HIV/AIDS are distributed unevenly across households, poverty may increase even if GDP per capita remains unchanged or even increases.
- Private and public spending on the response to HIV/AIDS absorbs resources which could otherwise be used for additional investment or consumption.
- The impact of and the response to HIV/AIDS affect government finance. If the economy grows more slowly as a consequence of HIV/AIDS, government revenues (but also certain expenses linked to the population size) also increase more slowly. The more direct implications of HIV/AIDS, though, are for government expenditures, as the response to HIV/AIDS absorbs fiscal resources. [...] HIV/AIDS [also] affects government spending beyond HIV/AIDS line items, through conditions like disability or orphanhood

addressed by non-HIV/AIDS specific spending, and through the costs of the impact of HIV/AIDS on government employees.

- HIV/AIDS affects the production costs of private enterprises, to the extent that increased morbidity affects the productivity of employees, or because of mortality-related disruptions. Early studies suggest that HIV/AIDS increases personnel costs by several percentage points in countries with high HIV prevalence.[36]

What makes HIV and AIDS a development issue for sub-Saharan Africa is not only or even primarily because it introduces large-scale economic impacts, much though these alter the life chances and prospects of individuals and communities in the worst-affected states. The larger point is that these outcomes combine with other structural and contextual matters—poverty especially—that shape and drive a range of further negative SRH outcomes in configurations of human suffering that are very difficult to break apart, prioritize and deal with.

Most immediately, although we can regard each instance of HIV infection as a failure of sexual health, the cumulative costs of dealing with the consequences also erode reproductive health, particularly non-HIV services for pregnant women and children.[37] In addition, because HIV infection compromises patients' immune systems, they become susceptible to opportunistic infections and co-morbidities, some of which often require difficult adjustments to antiretroviral treatment regimens. And the prevalence of non-HIV sexually transmitted diseases (STDs) in sub-Saharan Africa[38] multiplies the close links between sexual and reproductive health risk. 'Untreated or inappropriately treated, STDs may lead to severe complications, which account for most of their morbidity. Such complications occur most frequently in populations that lack ready access to effective treatment. Furthermore, both the anatomy of the female genital tract—prone to ascending infections—and reproductive events and related medical procedures—childbirth, stillbirth, abortion, uterine curettage and intrauterine device insertion—are additional risk factors for STD complications particular to women. The main STD complications include pelvic inflammatory disease and its sequelae, and the most important of these are impaired fertility and adverse pregnancy outcomes, enhanced HIV transmission, and cervical cancer.[39] In sub-Saharan Africa alone, 'an estimated 1,640,000 pregnant women have undiagnosed syphilis every year; almost all these women remain undetected.'[40]

The conditioning and facilitating context for these dynamics is pervasive poverty. Despite some impressive GDP growth statistics,[41] according to the World Bank, more than 40 per cent of sub-Saharan Africans live in poverty.[42] The persistence of poverty and inequality not only further worsens both sexual and reproductive health; it also exacerbates negative linkages between them, both directly and indirectly. So for example, food scarcity and malnourishment have dramatically worsened the number of stunted children in SSA (up from 45 million in 1990 to 57 million in 2015[43]), with maternal HIV status closely correlated with the stunted, underweight and wasted children.[44] Food insecurity also drives up the prevalence of risky, transactional sex and rates of non-adherence to antiretroviral medications.[45]

The other encompassing context for SRH in sub-Saharan Africa is its demography, which enlarges its scale and increases the urgency—again, with a strong gender slant. Currently, sub-Saharan Africa accounts for 90 per cent of AIDS-related adolescent deaths; and according to the United Nations Children's Fund (UNICEF), 'Three in four new HIV infections in adolescents (aged 15–19 years) occur in sub-Saharan Africa, and for every five adolescent boys living with HIV, there are seven girls (aged 10–19 years). This gender disparity grows as adolescents enter young adulthood. For every 5 young men living with HIV, there are 10 young women.'[46] Yet even as the sexually active population burgeons, there remains a great deal that we do now know about SSA adolescent risk and behaviour.[47] At the same time, the World Health Organization estimates 93 million new cases of STDs in SSA, with a range of serious risks for reproductive health including foetal and neonatal deaths arising from syphilis in pregnancy; human papillomavirus infection (HPV) facilitating cervical cancer; infertility resulting from gonorrhoea and chlamydia; and a three-fold increased risk of HIV infection in those with STDs such as syphilis.[48]

POLITICAL, NORMATIVE AND SOCIO-LEGAL PERSPECTIVES

There is no single perspective that can explain the rapid spread and persistence of sexual and reproductive health crises: biological, medical, interpersonal, psychological and cognitive, sociological—all are necessary, but none are sufficient on their own. However, to the degree that particular SRH issues present as public health crises nationally and regionally, there are further contexts which inform not only individuals' vulnerability, but also the permissibility of certain behaviours (which can either facilitate or inhibit them): perceptions of responsibility and blame; and constructions of broadly held, shared interests and values, expressed both formally (in law) and informally/normatively. These shape public responses, such as national health policy and health services priority-setting and the allocation of resources. And international expressions of interest, felt responsibility and a perceived need to build consensus as part of globalizing trends are hardly novel. For example, the *Programme of Action of the International Conference on Population and Development*,[49] held in Cairo in 1994 was itself a culmination of two decades of international consensus-building around sexual and reproductive health, explicitly framed as a development issue. The agreed *Programme of Action* explicitly brought sexual and reproductive health within the compass of already-established conventions and standards concerning the rights of individuals. Principle 8 stated:

> Everyone has the right to the enjoyment of the highest attainable standard of physical and mental health. States should take all appropriate measures to ensure, on a basis of equality of men and women, universal access to health-care services, including those related to reproductive health care, which includes family planning and sexual health. Reproductive health-care programmes should provide the widest range of services without any form of coercion. All couples and individuals have the basic right to decide freely and responsibly the number and spacing of their children and to have the information, education and means to do so.

Three sources of difficulty immediately ensued—and persist. The first is that (as will be discussed further in Chap. 3) to the extent that there is a serious state commitment to acknowledge sexual and reproductive health as a right, there is a greater willingness to deal with them as 'negatives'—that is, rights failures manifested as diseases and debilities, rather than as positive enhancements to the standing and autonomy of individuals (girls and women in especially) to make informed choices, to secure adequate protection from exploitation and coercion and to have affordable access to health services that will help them to secure their sexual and reproductive health. The second source of difficulty is that despite repeated, high-profile international and regional pronouncements, sexual and reproductive matters as rights remain controversial in many parts of the world—and in many parts of sub-Saharan Africa in particular. Political leaderships—even when they themselves subscribe to the principle—are acutely sensitive to dealing with sexual and reproductive health as rights and are cautious of provoking a normative backlash. And finally, when health resources are scarce, priorities tend to be skewed towards the urgencies of treatment rather than towards the more positive, preventive aspects of SRH. These points are captured in the following observation:

> Despite the obvious fact that sexual and reproductive ill health is a major cause of morbidity and mortality, with the exception of HIV and AIDS, the subject has failed to capture broad support from the donor community. Some argue that the notion of reproductive health that was promoted in Cairo was too idealistic, that by emphasising issues such as empowerment of women and reproductive rights rather than the provision of services and 'by asking too much, it ended up getting too little'. Others make the point that in the current climate of health sector reform, decisions to use scarce funding are based on the burden of death and disability attributable to a particular disorder on the basis of measures such as DALYs [Disability-Adjusted Life Year]. Sexual and reproductive health is not only about disease, but also about a collection of related health and human rights issues and many people are still confused about what it consists of. Furthermore, use of DALYs is not appropriate for quantification of the full burden of sexual and reproductive ill health. Pregnancy is not a disease, and associated complications are poorly counted unless they result in death; a stillbirth does not contribute even one DALY; reproductive morbidities are often inadequately measured and are generally under-reported because of associated stigma. Moreover, DALYs only measure death, disease, and disability without assigning any value to preventive interventions, such as family planning, that avoid ill health and promote well being, including in sexual matters.[50]

Of course, accessible, high-quality SRH services are clearly fundamental. But what necessarily precedes these is the bases upon which the nature and extent of all forms of medical care are determined—and this extends well beyond strictly biomedical realms. Since there is little that is random about vulnerability to disease (and still less about sexually transmitted ones), the obvious health vulnerabilities of adolescents and young adults arising from risky behaviours are shaped and amplified by the discriminatory and often pernicious ways in which gender relations are structured. Hence the Sustainable Development Goal 5 targets which include the elimination of all forms of discrimination against women and girls, including all forms of gender violence in the public and private spheres as well as harmful practices such as child, early and forced marriage and female genital mutilation—none of which come under the heading 'medical services.' Instead, these matters are relational. Rights (and the failure to recognize and enact them) are the thread that connects all levels of sexual and reproductive health—between sex partners, in respect of social responsibilities towards pregnant women, between citizens and state and between communities of identity and sexual preference. Rights restore the individual from aggregate statistics; establish the equal worth of all human lives; and they create the foundation for ensuring that the impulses of humane decency take the form of non-discriminatory, concerted action to ensure that they are enacted—and if need be, restored. For many, SRH rights remain contestable and even controversial. But they address the fundamentals of human health—that is, the *quality* of our relations at every level of human interaction and organization of political community. It is difficult to see how we might successfully combat the thicket of issues around SRH in sub-Saharan Africa without attending to the qualities of the forms of relatedness which give rise to and sustain them. It is to health rights that we now turn.

NOTES

1. Paul Farmer, *Infections and Inequalities: The Modern Plagues* (Oakland: University of California Press, 2001).
2. Jill Steans, and Daniela Tepe-Belfrage (eds), *Handbook of Gender in World Politics* (Oxford: Edward Elgar), 2016. See also: Juanita Elias and Adrienne Roberts, 'Feminist Global Political Economies of the Everyday: From Bingo to Bananas,' *Globalizations,* Vol. 13, No. 6 (2016), pp. 787–800.
3. See for example: A. A. Marphatia, T. J. Cole, C. Grijalva-Eterno and J.C.K. Wells, 'Associations of gender inequality with child malnutrition and mortality across 96 countries,' *Global Health, Epidemiology and Genomics, 1* (e6) (2016), https://doi.org/10.1017/gheg.2016.1
4. Paul Flowers, Graham Hart and Claire Marriott, 'Constructing Sexual Health: Gay Men and "Risk" in the Context of a Public Sex Environment,' *Journal of Health Psychology,* Vol. 4(4), (1999), p. 484.
5. Felicia Marie Knaul, et al., 'Rethinking maternal health,' *The Lancet Global Health,* Vol. 4, Issue 4 (22 April 2016), e227–28.
6. Ibid.
7. Steven Epstein and Laura Mamo, 'The proliferation of sexual health: Diverse social problems and the legitimation of sexuality,' *Social Sciences and Medicine,* Vol. 188 (September 2017), pp. 176–90.

8. UNFPA, Programme of Action adopted at the International Conference on Population and Development Cairo, 5–13 September 1994, p. 59. Available at: https://www.unfpa.org/sites/default/files/pub-pdf/programme_of_action_Web%20ENGLISH.pdf

9. For a chronological literature survey of definitions of sexual health, see Weston M. Edwards and Eli Coleman, 'Defining Sexual Health: A Descriptive Overview,' *Archives of Sexual Behavior*, Vol. 33, No. 3 (June 2004) pp. 189–195.

10. Available at: http://www.who.int/topics/sexual_health/en/

11. Mark Golden and Peter Toohey (eds), *A cultural history of sexuality in the classical world* (Oxford: Berg, 2011); Matthew Sommer, *Sex, Law and Society in Late Imperial China* (Stanford: Stanford University Press, 2000); Ze'ev Maghen, *Virtues of the Flesh: Passion and Purity in Early Islamic Jurisprudence* (Leiden: Brill, 2005).

12. Mary Douglas, *Purity and Danger: An Analysis of the Concept of Pollution and Taboo* (London: Routledge, 2002).

13. Nana K. Poku and Jesper Sundewall, 'Political responsibility and global health,' *Third World Quarterly*, DOI: https://doi.org/10.1080/0143659 7.2017.1369034

14. John Stove et al., 'What Is Required to End the AIDS Epidemic as a Public Health Threat by 2030? The Cost and Impact of the Fast-Track Approach,' *PLoS ONE* 11(5) (2016), e0154893. doi:10.1371/journal.pone.0154893; Jon Cohen, 'South Africa's bid to end AIDS,' *Science*, Vol. 353 (6294) (1 July 2016), pp. 18–21.

15. See for example: Geoff Foster, Carol Levine, and John Williamson (eds), *A generation at risk: the global impact of HIV/AIDS on orphans and vulnerable children* (Cambridge: Cambridge University Press, 2005).

16. P. Allotey and D. D. Reidpath, 'Sexual and reproductive health and rights post 2015—challenges and opportunities,' *BJOG*, Vol. 122, Issue 2 (January 2015), p. 152. See also: World Health Organization, *Global and Regional Estimates of Violence Against Women: Prevalence and Health Effects of Intimate Partner Violence and non-Partner Sexual Violence*. Geneva: World Health Organisation, 2013. Available at: www.who.int/reproductivehealth/publications/violence/9789241564625/en/

17. Ibid.

18. Anna Glasier, A. Metin Gülmezoglu, George P. Schmid, Claudia Garcia-Moreno, Paul FA Van Look, 'Sexual and reproductive health: a matter of life and death,' *Lancet* 368 (2006), 1595–607 (quoted passage not numbered).

19. According to the UN's *Millennium Development Goals Report* (2015), 'Official development assistance from developed countries increased 66 percent in real terms from 2000 and 2014, reaching $135.2 billion.'

20. Alicia Ely Yamin and Vanessa M. Boulanger, 'Why Global Goals and Indicators Matter: the Experience of Sexual and Reproductive Health and Rights in the Millennium Development Goals,' *Journal of Human Development and Capabilities*, Vol. 15, Issues 2–3 (April 2014), pp. 1–14.

21. IPFF, UNFPA and WHO, *SRH and HIV Linkages Compendium: Indicators and Related Assessment Tools* (2014). Available at: http://srh-hivlinkages.org/wp-content/uploads/SRH-HIV-Linkages-Compendium_rev.pdf

22. See for example: UNFPA, Glion Call to Action on Family Planning and HIV/AIDS in Women and Children (2004), available at: https://www.k4health.org/sites/default/files/Glion%20Call%20to%20Action.pdf

23. Sabina A. Haberlen, Manjulaa Narasimhan, Laura K. Beres, and Caitlin E. Kennedy, 'Integration of Family Planning Services into HIV Care and Treatment Services: A Systematic Review,' *Studies in Family Planning* 48(2), (2017), pp. 153–77; Charlotte E. Warren, Susannah H. Mayhew and Jonathan Hopkins, 'The Current Status of Research on the Integration of Sexual and Reproductive Health and HIV Services,' *Studies in Family Planning* 48(2), (2017), pp. 91–105.

24. H. A. Gesesew et al., 'Significant association between perceived HIV related stigma and late presentation for HIV/AIDS care in low and middle-income countries: A systematic review and meta-analysis,' *PLoS ONE* 12(3): e0173928. Available at: https://doi.org/10.1371/journal.pone.0173928

25. Sharon Fonn and TK Sundari Ravindran, 'The macroeconomic environment and sexual and reproductive health: a review of trends over the last 30 years,' *Reproductive Health Matters*, Vol. 19, No. 38 (November 2011), pp. 11–25.

26. According to the World Bank, 'The world's Middle Income Countries (MICs), which are defined as having a per capita gross national income of US$1,026 to $12,475 (2011) are a diverse group by size, population, and income level. Middle income countries are home to five of the world's seven billion people and 73 per cent of the world's poor people. At the same time, middle income countries represent about one third of global GDP and are major engines of global growth.' http://www.worldbank.org/en/country/mic/overview; see also: Channing Arndt, Andy McKay, and Finn Tarp (eds), *Growth and Poverty in Sub Saharan* Africa, A study prepared by the United Nations University World Institute for Development Economics Research (Oxford: Oxford University Press, 2016).

27. Andy Sumner, 'Global Poverty and the New Bottom Billion: What if Three-quarters of the World's Poor Live in Middle-income Countries?' IDS Working paper 349 (November 2010).

28. David Canning, Sangeeta Raja, and Abdo S. Yazbeck (eds), *Africa's Demographic Transition: Dividend or Disaster?* (A co-publication of Agence Française de Développement and the World Bank) (2015). Available at: https://openknowledge.worldbank.org/bitstream/handle/10986/22036/AfrDemographicTransitionOVERVIEW.pdf?sequence=5&isAllowed=y

29. Nick Goulding et al., 'Mapping under-5 and neonatal mortality in Africa, 2000–15: a baseline analysis for the Sustainable Development Goals,' *The Lancet*, Vol. 390, No. 10108 (11 November 2017), pp. 2171–82.

30. World Health Statistics data visualizations dashboard, available at: http://apps.who.int/gho/data/view.sdg.3-2-data-reg?lang=en

31. World Health Organization, Universal health Care data Portal, available at: http://apps.who.int/gho/cabinet/uhc-service-coverage.jsp

32. Marni Sommer and Kristin Mmari, 'Addressing Structural and Environmental Factors for Adolescent Sexual and Reproductive Health in Low- and Middle-Income Countries,' *American Journal of Public Health* Vol. 105, No. 10 (October 2015), pp. 1973–81.

33. United Nations Development Programme, *Africa Human Development Report, 2016: Accelerating Gender Equality and Women's Empowerment in Africa*, available at: http://www.undp.org/content/undp/en/home/librarypage/hdr/2016-africa-human-development-report.html

34. United Nations Population Fund, available at: https://www.unfpa.org/hiv-aids

35. United Nations Population Fund (UNFPA), available at: https://www.unfpa.org/hiv-aids

36. Markus Haacker, *The Economics of the Global Response to HIV/AIDS* (Oxford: Oxford University Press, 2016), pp. 50–1.

37. Anne Case and Christina Paxson, 'The Impact of the AIDS Pandemic on Health Services in Africa: Evidence from Demographic and Health Surveys,' *Demography* Vol. 48, Issue 2 (2011), pp. 675–91.

38. Elizabeth A. Torrone, 'Prevalence of sexually transmitted infections and bacterial vaginosis among women in sub-Saharan Africa: An individual participant data meta-analysis of 18 HIV prevention studies,' *PLOS Medicine* (27 February 2018), https://doi.org/10.1371/journal.pmed.1002511

39. Institute of Medicine and Christopher P. Howson, *In Her Lifetime: Female Morbidity and Mortality in Sub-Saharan Africa* (Washington, D.C.: National Academies Press, 1996), p. 244.

40. Anna Glasier et al., 'Sexual and reproductive health: a matter of life and death' The *Lancet*, 368, Vol. 9547 (2006), p. 1600.

41. Channing Arndt, Andy McKay, and Finn Tarp (eds), *Growth and Poverty in Sub Saharan Africa*, A study prepared by the United Nations University

World Institute for Development Economics Research (Oxford: Oxford University Press, 2016).

42. Kathleen Beegle, Luc Christiaensen Andrew Dabalen Isis Gaddis, *Poverty in a Rising Africa* (Washington, D.C.: The World Bank, 2016).

43. World Bank, World in Review: 2017. Available at: http://www.world-bank.org/en/news/feature/2017/12/15/year-in-review-2017-in-12-charts

44. Monica A. Magad, 'Household and community HIV/AIDS status and child malnutrition in sub-Saharan Africa: Evidence from the demographic and health surveys,' *Social Science & Medicine*, Vol. 73, Issue, (August 2011), pp. 436–46.

45. Elisabeth Chop et al., 'Food insecurity, sexual risk behavior, and adherence to antiretroviral therapy among women living with HIV: A systematic review,' *Health Care for Women International*, 38(9) (2017), pp. 927–44.

46. https://data.unicef.org/wp-content/uploads/2017/11/HIVAIDS-Statistical-Update-2017.pdf

47. See for example: Elona Toska et al., 'Sex in the shadow of HIV: A systematic review of prevalence, risk factors, and interventions to reduce sexual risk-taking among HIV positive adolescents and youth in sub- Saharan Africa,' *PLoS One*, Vol. 12, No. 6 (June 2017); Rachel Kidman and Philip Anglewicz, 'Are adolescent orphans more likely to be HIV-positive? A pooled data analyses across 19 countries in sub-Saharan Africa,' *Journal of Epidemiology and Community Health*, Vol. 70, Issue 8 (August 2016), p. 795.

48. http://apps.who.int/iris/bitstream/handle/10665/82207/WHO_RHR_13.02_eng.pdf;jsessionid=8349B401BC5772DB7C808346AF806 8B5?sequence=1

49. Programme of Action of the International Conference on Population and development, 5–13 September 1994. Available at: https://www.unfpa.org/sites/default/files/pub-pdf/programme_of_action_Web%20 ENGLISH.pdf

50. Anna Glasier et al., op cit., p. 1604.

CHAPTER 3

Sexual and Reproductive Health as Rights

Abstract The first section opens with an introduction to the fundamental sources of contention around human rights, particularly as they apply to human health. This is followed by an outline of the status of key human rights treaties in the context of sexual and reproductive health in sub-Saharan Africa. A human right to health is then contrasted with citizen entitlements. An integrated conception of sexual and reproductive health is set out in detail, tracing the development of reproductive health from a stand-alone health matter detached from sexual rights to conceptions where the two are viewed as necessarily joined.

Keywords Human rights • Norms • Laws • Citizen entitlements

HUMAN RIGHTS

Historically, the idea and ideal of human rights was and remains a culmination of the age-old struggle of peoples everywhere, in every century to assert the fundamental and equal worth of every human being against the prerogatives of power. Another way of expressing this is to say that human rights make every relationship of absolute power anathema: we cannot have a human rights regime *and* slavery, torture or wanton slaughter.

© The Author(s), under exclusive license to Springer Nature Singapore Pte Ltd. 2020
N. K. Poku, *Sexual and Reproductive Health and Rights in Sub-Saharan Africa*, Global Research in Gender, Sexuality and Health, https://doi.org/10.1007/978-981-15-8502-9_3

Human rights are inherently political because they assert a limit to the accrual and exercise of power—and for that reason, they are never finally and completely won—but nor are they entirely aspirational, since they are now deeply entrenched within international and national law.[1] Human rights are generally regarded as having the following characteristics:

- They apply universally to all human beings;
- They are inalienable—they cannot be granted or revoked, bought, sold or given away;
- Human rights are paramount—that is, they are not trivial; we cannot deprive someone of their rights without a grave affront to justice;
- Human rights claims ought to be practicable and realizable for all; and
- Human rights must be effective/enforceable.

The legal standing of human rights, beginning with the Universal Declaration in 1948 has not supplanted legal, political and philosophical arguments about whether and how they can be 'grounded'; and the contested boundaries between what counts as a human right and a citizen entitlement are now a fixture of politico-legal life in most countries. But what concerns us here is that states and the international system have incorporated them in law; and after 70 years, there is now a great deal of normative expectation of respect for fundamental human rights, to the degree that states which grossly abuse the human rights of their citizens are deemed to have compromised their sovereign integrity, opening the way for legally sanctioned intervention.[2]

Although Article 25(i) of Universal Declaration of Human Rights states that '[e]veryone has the right to a standard of living adequate for the health and well-being of himself and of his [sic] family, including food, clothing, housing and medical care and necessary social services, and the right to security in the event of unemployment, sickness, disability, widowhood, old age or lack of livelihood in circumstances beyond their control,'[3] health as a human right remains contested. In 1999, exchanges over the right to health were conducted in the *British Medical Journal*, a publication that has a long history of concern over human rights.[4] Opening the debate, the Tavistock Group offered a draft for a set of ethical principles that affirmed the human right to health. The draft sought to provide a basis for discussion among all branches of the medical and health care professions that would, the authors hoped, end in a general agreement on the nature of a right to health.

The fundamental principle underscoring the proposal was that while rights are the possessions of individuals, the community has a duty to fulfil those rights. Accordingly, as a human right, the right to health cannot be bought and sold in the market place like other commodities. Nor can the right to health be limited by the ability to pay. Instead, the proposal argued that governments and the wider international community have an obligation to fund medical education, training and research, to make provision for sustainable investment in support of health care professionals and to ensure that knowledge is exchanged freely and without regard for institutional or national affiliations and claims to ownership.[5] The responses to this proposal drew upon well-known liberal objections to a right to health. Liberal arguments against accepting a right to health as a human right rest upon the presumption that civil and political rights are qualitatively and significantly different from socio-economic rights. This distinction is usually expressed as being between 'negative' rights (civil and political) and 'positive' rights (economic, social and cultural). Although not expressed explicitly in these terms, disagreements over negative versus positive rights are at the heart of the debate conducted in the *British Medical Journal*.

Following this positive/negative distinction, it is frequently argued that negative rights are fulfilled when all members of a community exercise restraint from doing anything that might violate the freedoms of others to pursue their own interests. While liberals reject the libertarian conclusions that this approach to rights might suggest, negative freedoms can be legitimately constrained only in the interests of all members of the community enjoying an equal right to civil and political liberties. Positive rights, on the other hand, require others to provide the material means of life and security to those unable to provide for themselves: at a minimum, clean water, shelter, food and health care.[6] While the protection of negative rights demands nothing more than forbearance, the protection of positive rights demands social organization for redistributing resources.

Briefly, the defence of negative claims against the more expansive claims of positive one rests upon the following logic[7]: Negative rights can be guaranteed in law, whereas positive rights cannot—the 'fact that there is no scarcity consideration makes [negative rights] justiciable and capable of being fully respected and implemented because it consists of forbearance rather than action.'[8] Furthermore, the guarantee of positive rights depends upon a country's level of economic development, so no universal standard can be applied. Thus, while negative rights imply 'can' positive rights imply 'ought' and are therefore qualitatively distinct.[9] Proponents of negative rights also assert that positive rights are culturally determined, and cannot therefore be considered as universal claims,[10] and that there is no duty holder for positive rights, whereas forbearance is a duty held by all. On this line of reasoning, any individual's health is the result of physical and biological processes, and/or good or bad luck, for neither of which others can be held liable. Finally, the champions of negative over positive rights observe that since negative rights are the rights we claim as individuals, and economic and social rights are rights dependent upon community and social policy, positive rights cannot be understood as human rights, but rather as citizen entitlements, which vary from state to state. Since negative rights are the rights we claim as individuals, and economic and social rights are rights dependent upon community and social policy, positive rights cannot be regarded as human rights.

In response to these liberal arguments, it might be argued that neither rights to physical security nor socio-economic rights 'fit neatly into their assigned sides of the simplistic positive/negative dichotomy.'[11] Henry Shue argues that there are three rights, without which no other rights can be enjoyed. These are the rights to life, security and subsistence, where subsistence is understood to include the means to sustain physical and social life, including the right to health. For Shue, none of these claims is wholly positive or negative. For example, while in some cases it is correct to understand physical security as a negative right, in the sense that all members of society have a duty of forbearance, this is only a partial description of what we understand by human rights. According to this argument, even liberals must accept that the right to security implies something more than forbearance, namely the need to make social arrangements to protect actively those whose security is threatened. The demand for civil and political rights is 'not normally a demand simply to be left alone, but a demand to be protected against harm ... It is a demand for positive action ... a demand for social guarantees against at least the standard threats.'[12] From this perspective, liberal claims that real rights demand merely forbearance overlook the necessity for state intervention in the name of protecting those human rights, for example, taxation to fund a legislature, police force, legal system, courts and prisons. Furthermore, if there are costs attached to both negative and positive rights, and we can reach a consensus on an acceptable level of expenditure for protecting civil and political rights, then why not for socio-economic rights?[13]

Similarly, socio-economic rights can often be guaranteed through forbearance, in the sense that the actions of others often act as a barrier that limits people's capabilities to help themselves. As Shue expresses it,

> All that is sometimes necessary is to protect the persons whose subsistence is threatened from the individuals and institutions that will otherwise intentionally or unintentionally harm them. A demand for a right to subsistence may involve not a demand to be provided with grants of commodities but merely a demand to be provided some opportunity for supporting oneself. The request is not to be supported but to be allowed to be self-supporting on the basis of one's own hard work.[14]

This implies that if legal, economic, social and policy barriers deny people an opportunity to gain access to the necessary resources to secure their own basic rights then this should be understood as a violation of universal human rights. Under conditions of globalization, where the quality of life is determined by a wide range of institutions (regional, global as well as regional and national), this conclusion has far-reaching consequences for securing the health of peoples everywhere, including those least able to provide for themselves.

Clearly, procuring and defending negative human rights are different in character from enacting positive ones for reasons that include but extend beyond philosophical ones; nevertheless, the practical and moral awfulness of our countless failures to enact positive human rights—in health not least—stand in stark contrast to the importance that states assign to negative ones.

This disparity was expressed in direct terms by the UN Committee on Economic, Social and Cultural Rights in its statement to the Vienna World Conference of 1993:

> The shocking reality ... is that states and the international community as a whole continue to tolerate all too often breaches of economic, social and cultural rights which, if they occurred in relation to civil and political rights, would provoke expressions of horror and outrage and would lead to concerted calls for immediate remedial action. In effect, despite the rhetoric, violations of civil and political rights continue to be treated as though they were far more serious, and more patently intolerable, than massive and direct denials of economic, social and cultural rights.[15]

The reason why states are nevertheless at least nominally committed to positive human rights (including the right to health) is distinct from but closely related to their often faltering commitment to negative rights. The instigation and development of human rights is part of a much longer history of slow, often painful realignments of power relations between governments and people—that is, the idea of legitimacy as something other than divinely ordained or taken and held by brute force. And as democracy as an idea and ideal took hold, so too did the expectation of state responsibilities towards their citizens and the development of mechanisms of accountability. Over time, this has come to include at least basic social welfare provision, which plainly encompasses the fundamentals of human health—the rapid pace of population growth and urbanization adding considerable self-interested impetus.[16] In view of the number and severity of human rights violations since the inauguration of the Universal Declaration in 1948, and the continuance of preventable human suffering on unconscionable scales, it would be easy to dismiss human rights law as largely a 'dead letter'—optional at best and dismissible when not in conformity with state interests because they cannot be enforced. Yet that would overlook the power of norms—the lived expectations of peoples everywhere, together with the expectations of states themselves within an evolving international system.[17] Normative expectation within the international system is not only at the root of the Responsibility to Protect[18] which provides a means of redress for gross violations of negative human rights: similar pressures, both between and within states, are now operative in positive human rights, too—and most notably in the field of health.

We can see this is both the Millennium Development Goals (MDGs, 2000–15) and the current Sustainable Development Goals (SDGs). The point is not merely that four of the eight MDGs focused directly or indirectly on health,[19] but that health issues (and in particular, the health of women) were explicitly brought into national and international political arenas. Of course,

> [t]he MDGs [did] not (and could not) make an explicit link between international organisation and poverty. This is not a fatal flaw, but reflects the power of state interests and institutional momentum in ways that also apply to the advancement of positive human rights. By dint of their standing and inclusiveness, the MDGs [brought] into focus structural disadvantages, inequitable relations and contradictions between professed ideals and countervailing expressions of self-interest. This is a thin reed, but it is not

worthless; it is a feature the MDGs share[d] with the human rights regime: the potential of norm diffusion and embedding to edge the powerful beyond what deliberative self-interest would otherwise entertain.[20]

There are many drivers for changes in normative expectations around health: increasingly visible gross disparities in the life chances of large populations both within and between societies; the means to prevent, cure or alleviate many of the long-standing scourges of humanity—often at very low cost, including preventive measures such as the provision of safe drinking water, adequate sanitation and childhood nutrition; the demand that democratically elected governments behave responsibly and responsively; and the threats posed to social coherence by widespread disease and debility—matters neither entirely historical nor confined to HIV/AIDS.[21] The human rights regime speaks to all of these matters and more: it strengthens normative expectation around particular issues and in turn gains strength as an engine for the advancement of human equality. For example, a lawsuit brought against the government of South Africa by a consortium of 40 pharmaceutical companies (initially with the backing of their home governments) against a law that allowed generic substitution of AIDS medicines faced vociferous worldwide resistance and eventually collapsed because 'by the time the case finally reached the courtroom in May 2000, the drug companies could no longer count on the support of their home governments. Demonstrators in major cities asked the companies to drop the case; [and] several governments and parliaments around the world, including the European Parliament, demanded that the companies withdraw from the case. The legal action turned into a public relations disaster for the drug companies.'[22] This led to the Doha Agreement for the legal manufacture of affordable, generic antiretrovirals for AIDS treatment and the saving of millions of lives.

In addition to an enduring negative/positive rights split breaking down before the logical point that negative freedoms cannot be enjoyed without a modicum of health, there is also a range of pragmatic and values-driven considerations that further undermine it—that gross inequities in health are a challenge to social coherence and an affront to the shared values meant to be upheld by negative rights; and that weakly grounded, piecemeal citizen entitlements to health care are inadequate to the scale of the need, worldwide. 'Recent World Bank/World Health Organization (WHO) research from 2017 shows that half the world's population cannot access needed health services, while 100 million people are pushed into extreme poverty each year because of health expenses. In addition, 800 million people spend at least 10 per cent or more of their household budget on healthcare expenses.'[23]

Despite this state of affairs, the enshrinement of positive human rights in international covenants to which the majority of sub-Saharan countries have subscribed is impressive—all the more given those specific to the continent. Indeed, Article 14 of the African Women's Protocol (AWP) to the African Charter on Human and Peoples' Rights[24] is devoted specifically to health and reproductive rights (albeit with the specifics of sexual health noticeably absent) and includes the right of women to control their fertility; to decide whether to have children, their number and spacing; to choose any method of contraception; to have family planning education; and to protect the reproductive rights of women by authorizing medical abortion in cases of sexual assault, rape, incest and where the continued pregnancy endangers the mental and physical health of the mother or the life of the mother or the foetus. While by no means covering the full extent of sexual and reproductive health (SRH), it is nevertheless a remarkable commitment, especially when set beside the scale of the need (Table 3.1).

Table 3.1 Status of key human rights treaties in the context of SRH in sub-Saharan Africa

African Charter on Human and Peoples' Rights (ACHPR)	African Women's Protocol (AWP)	International Covenants on Civil and Political Rights (ICCPR)	International Covenant on Economic, Social and Cultural Rights (ICESCR)	Convention on the Elimination of All Forms of Discrimination Against Women (CEDAW)
The only African state that has not signed and ratified the Charter is South Sudan	28 member states of the African Union have signed and ratified the AWP; 19 have signed but not ratified; and 4 states have not signed: Botswana, Egypt, Eritrea and Tunisia	172 states are party to the ICCPR, including all sub-Saharan African states, with the exception of South Sudan	169 countries are party to the ICESCR. The only African states that have neither signed nor ratified the Convention are Botswana, Mozambique and South Sudan [the United States has signed but not ratified the Convention]	Only five states have not ratified CEDAW, two of them in sub-Saharan Africa: Somalia and Sudan

However, only just over half of African Union states have both signed and ratified the African Women's protocol; and even the near-comprehensive assent of states to the primary covenants for positive human rights (the International Covenant on Civil and Political Rights or ICCPR and International Covenant on Economic, Social and Cultural Rights or ICESCR) appear to have more rhetorical force than practical effect. The same holds for the Convention on the Elimination of Discrimination Against Women (CEDAW). In addition, the Maputo Protocol to the African Charter on Human and Peoples' Rights (ACHPR) has been adopted by all but three of the African Union's (AU's) member states; and while section 14 of the Protocol addresses 'Health and Reproductive Rights,' it leaves out sexual rights or any explicit use of the term 'human rights.'

Yet these disappointments do not render the enshrinement of human rights either as a principle or in any of its particulars a cynical exercise or a dead letter. Both within and between states, norms and laws relate to each other in complex configurations and at incongruent speeds (which is why it takes a brave politician to advocate legal change which is out of synch with established norms). Most laws are enacted rather than enforced because they consolidate or express changed and changing social norms. But this does not mean that writing forward-looking legal instruments to establish and specify human rights is done in the misplaced hope that international covenants will be immediately transformative—after all, even on an assumption of good faith by all states party to positive human rights conventions, the commitment of the poorest could fairly be regarded as aspirational. It is notable that the substance of the Millennium Development Goals fell squarely within long-standing commitments to positive human rights, but in the Millennium Declaration of 2000, the deployment of 'human rights' in the document was sparing—only eight mentions, largely in language familiar since the 1948 Universal Declaration of Human Rights.[25] States maintain an ambivalent attitude towards enshrining positive human rights, yet they are generally sensitive to the health needs of their populations, if only for practical reasons. It would be a thin conceptualization of 'development' that did not include at least basic health care provision.

It is very difficult to determine the effectiveness of these and related conventions. This is because tracing causal dynamics arising from a health-related human rights convention are vexed when key sexual and reproductive health indicators are subject to a very wide range of interconnected socio-economic and socio-cultural variables[26]—a point implicit in the provisions of both the ICCPR and the ICESCR. In one large-scale study using data from 194 countries against 72 key indicators, the researchers concluded that the status of treaty ratification alone is not a good indicator of the realization of the right to health.[27] This is hardly surprising given that normative conformity is attractive for states, particularly when non-adherence to enactment and reporting provisions risk little in the way of sanctions or opprobrium—a point central to the larger panoply of positive human rights. Moreover, a systematic study of all the world's national constitutions '… analysed the full range of ways that broad health rights can be guaranteed [and] found that 86 countries (45 per cent) did not guarantee their citizens any kind of health protection.' The breakdown is still less heartening:

> In international conventions and agreements, health protection is articulated as a right both to public health or preventative measures and to medical care services. With respect to these specific rights, the status of the world's constitutions can be described as either half empty or half full. Seventy-three countries (38 per cent) guaranteed the right to medical care services and another 27 (14 per cent) aspired to protect this right in 2011. Nine per cent of countries provided a constitutionally guaranteed right to free health care. When it came to guaranteeing public health, the global performance was poorer. Only 27 countries (14 per cent) guaranteed this right, and 21 (11 per cent) aspired to it.[28]

There is no single pathway or dynamic by which those human rights to health already enshrined in international covenants can be realized, or in some cases commenced, but some combination of both popular and international norms, the slow entrenchment of 'good governance' criteria, economic growth in less developed economies, the pressure of HIV/AIDS as a phenomenon which cuts across discrete health issue boundaries as well as across national borders and a growing movement dedicated to fundamental health improvements globally (the Millennium Development and Sustainable Development Goals; the impetus to establish Universal Health Coverage (UHC))[29] all play a part. Enactment of the universality and clarity of international covenants covering the human right to health are at best uncertain, sparse and gradualist, even though, as we have seen, the case for abstracting positive from negative human rights in conditions where millions struggle to survive is not credible.[30]

In any event, the pathways between human rights, international decla-rations of a right to health and their enactment within national jurisdic-tions are never as linear as the formal commitments might suggest. For example, in that region of the world where the human rights regime is longest and arguably most deeply embedded in both national and interna-tional statutes, the European Union (EU), whose member states also enjoy highly developed and generally accessible health services, has its own lego-political complexities in giving expression to agreed legal principles; coordinating clearly connected but not explicitly acknowledged connec-tions between a right to health and disparate health and health-related issue areas; grappling with the jurisprudential and political implications of enactments or failures to enact; and harmonizing national against com-munity interests and capacities. To cite but one example:

> Article 35 [of the Charter of Fundamental Rights of the European Union], on the 'right to health'[31] is part of EU law. [...] The EU and the Member States share responsibility for several policy areas which clearly connect to the 'right to health'. These include environmental policy, food regulation, tobacco regulation, and access to timely provision of health care services, at least in a cross-border context. And yet, the institutions of the EU appear, in virtually all cases, to have studiously ignored the connection between the 'right to health' as developed by the 'jurisprudence' under the [European Social Charter], and various relevant EU policies.[32]

Although declarations of a human right to health in international cov-enants often signal little more than normative conformity at a formal level, insufficient on its own for practical purposes, they are nevertheless neces-sary as a means of recasting a great deal of ill health not as part of the human condition but as political matters potentially subject to redress. And although the philosophical tension between health rights and entitle-ments is essentially unresolvable,[33] that does not preclude either an enlargement of the compass of rights or their enactment. And normative congruence with improvements in health provisions, however they come about, can be an effective solvent for philosophical contention, particu-larly when the fundamentals for survival and pain-free lives are at stake. At the same time, however, progress is not inevitable; and norm regress, even in some of the fundamentals of human rights, has already occurred.[34]

Outside the compass of rights (both human rights and citizen entitle-ments) individuals and groups can receive forms and degrees of health care—in emergency situations, by dint of international largesse or charitable initiatives and indirectly, through various kinds of developmental or infrastructural improvements to the conditions in which the poorest and least healthy live and work. However, these are often short-term, intermittent, do not always take account of access/affordability issues and are subject to shifting political priorities. In the absence of a right to health, health services are subject to the ability to pay—and for many millions, even the bare minimum is beyond their reach. The human right to health is catalytic, not transformative, and political engagement with the obligations to which nearly every nation has subscribed, however this comes about, opens up pathways to the attainment of health for many millions as a matter of public policy and not merely private aspiration for those currently disenfranchised. In any event, demarcations between international and domestic law, between formal obligations and social norms, and between unassailable rights and conditional entitlements are less binary than the categories suggest. Moreover, political, legal and social dynamics variously progress and/or inhibit the attainment of health and its myriad components in ways that sometimes cut across discrete institutional and professional arenas, such as the protests that eventuated in the Doha Agreement (recounted above).

The uniqueness of human rights (including the human right to health) is that they are universal and inalienable. All other forms of law-based rights or constitutionally prescribed citizen entitlements are conditional—that is, they are variously limited in their scope or application, at times by dint of being congruent with restrictive or repressive laws, such as punitive statutes against homosexuality. Furthermore, while illegal behaviours or criminal convictions do not deprive men and women of their human rights (and for the purposes of SRH, this notably includes sex workers, drug users and prisoners), they often preclude those individuals from seeking as well as accessing SRH services as part of nationally sanctioned and funded health services.

Clearly, neither citizen rights nor human rights can vault over political contention, but they do powerfully frame and shape it.

The narrative of how human rights language has been appropriated, more and less effectively, by different social actors and movements (including in the domain of health) underscores how rights and paradigms of rights are not self-standing truths, but loci of contestation over power. Rights are terse formulations of profound arguments about distributive justice and humanity. If we seek to use rights to promote social justice in health, it is a strategic mistake to think that merely using the short-hand is enough to circumvent the argument.[35]

CITIZEN ENTITLEMENTS

The logic and empathetic responsiveness of enabling a right to health is compelling, and at the national-constitutional level it is hardly radical—nearly half of the world's countries have some forms and degrees of a right to health for their citizens. But within sub-Saharan Africa no less than the rest of the world, the extent of constitutionally guaranteed rights to health is often characterized by high ideals lacking specifics and/or by striking omissions. For instance, despite the AWP, no African constitution refers to the importance of making free and autonomous sexual and reproductive rights decisions; and worldwide, only five states do.[36] And what is true about the right to health generally is starkly true of sexual and reproductive health rights, as the continuance of the AIDS pandemic attests.

However, one notable manner in which governments which preside over inadequately provisioned or un-enacted constitutional and national health laws can be prompted to action is through national courts. There are times when a formally acknowledged and legally encoded human right to health can be deployed instrumentally[37] in order to hold governments to account and/or to mobilize citizenry[38] in sufficient numbers to edge legal principles into lego-political arenas and to undertake legal action. The legal and political arenas meet at the point of justiciability, and the best-established pathway to securing health rights is through litigation.

In many ways, the advent of effective antiretroviral medications (ARVs) in the mid-1990s spawned much of the later health rights litigation. Clear linkages to the right to life, coupled often with issues of discrimination against marginalized groups, and the existence of a clearly defined remedy all contributed to the framing of enforceable legal claims. In the case of AIDS treatment, the existence of important social movements strengthened demands for ARVs in terms of rights, as well as implementation of legal judgements, when many political branches of government had previously shown indifference or resistance to providing treatment for people living with HIV/AIDS.

For example, in 2001, the '[South African HIV and AIDS] Treatment Action Campaign brought a suit against the South African government, alleging that its restrictions on the availability of [AIDS drug] Nevirapine (limiting it in the public sector to hospitals involved in a pilot study) and its failure to have a reasonable plan to make the drug more widely available violated the right to health of HIV-positive pregnant women and their children guaranteed in the South African constitution.'[39] The finding in favour of the claimants was upheld in the Constitutional Court of South Africa, based on the provisions of the country's post-apartheid constitution, Section 27 of which states, '(1) Everyone has the right to have access to (a) health care services, including reproductive health care; (b) sufficient food and water; and (c) social security ... (2) The state must take reasonable legislative and other measures, within its available resources, to achieve the progressive realization of each of these rights.'

Since then, health rights litigation has expanded to many other topics and has begun to have a substantial impact in countries across the world, affecting tens of thousands of individual entitlements to medications and treatments a year in some countries, but also rewriting intellectual property rules, ensuring regulation of laws, causing changes in policies of various kinds, and influencing health priority-setting processes and budgetary allocations.[40] National courts also have a vital role in addressing the health obligations of states towards their citizens, often in ways which tacitly acknowledge the negative/positive human rights dichotomy, but not as a fixed impediment to the progressive implementation positive human rights.[41]

INTEGRATED CONCEPTION OF SEXUAL AND REPRODUCTIVE HEALTH

Beyond the universal requisites for survival, perhaps no aspect of human health or the conditions which enable it can be deemed 'most fundamental' for every purpose. Epidemic and pandemic health emergencies, large-scale preventive initiatives such as inoculation programmes and population-level vulnerabilities all present as fundamental and urgent; so do worrying combinations of demographic indicators combined with disease trends. But sexual and reproductive health is more than a health 'hardy perennial': it is truly at the base of human continuance and flourishing—in every nation and at every scale, from population growth and the earth's carrying capacity[42] to the social mores that shape gender and sexual conduct. And sexual and reproductive health is unique in that it combines the most personal, intimate and powerful human urges with meanings and outcomes that are also enduringly socio-cultural and political—and even environmental. SRH therefore extends far beyond the medically-specific bounds of disease prevention and treatment, or the management of the procreative cycle because in matters sexual and reproductive, the corporeal, the relational and the political can never be fully abstracted from one another, as the authors of a comprehensive literature survey of the meanings of 'sexual health' discovered, identifying the following themes:

> Containing the spread of sexually transmitted infections; addressing failures of sexual functioning; controlling population growth and promoting procreative autonomy; solving injustices linked to the absence of sexual rights; [and] containing threats of irresponsible sexual behavior.[43]

The authors conclude:

> While sexual health certainly includes narrowly biomedical or public health-related preoccupations with matters such as risk and surveillance, it also provides a cloak of legitimacy to a range of sexuality-related concerns—pleasure, rights, autonomy, freedom, desire—not currently inscribed as biomedical. [F]urther work is needed to explore and understand the various ways by which sexuality is made an object of attention as part of a more widespread will to health. Among other things, such analysis should aim to locate sexuality in its intersections with social class, gender, and race, and should place these intersections within the broader political, cultural, and social contexts in which individuals are enjoined to seek health, wellness, and fitness and lead responsible lives.[44]

Much the same applies to reproductive health: few of its meanings can be engaged without a consideration of personhood and agency, or an awareness of the contexts which shape both health behaviours and outcomes—policies, health systems, social norms (particularly with respect to gender) and the full range of socio-economic indicators that have a powerful bearing on reproductive options and choices, where they exist. More than any other field in medicine, sexual and reproductive health are inescapably relational—and not merely to each other: even for medical purposes, they cannot be reduced to the biomedical particulars of bodies. These and similar conceptions of sexual and reproductive health find consolidated expression in the Guttmacher-Lancet Commission report.

DEFINING SEXUAL AND REPRODUCTIVE HEALTH

The most comprehensive and detailed delineation of sexual and reproductive health was produced by the Guttmacher-Lancet Commission in 2018.[45] For all of the substance and precision devoted to defining SRH, together with a consideration of contexts and determinants, the purpose and orientation of the report is dedicated to specifying and advocating a rights-based approach to the achievement of SRH for all. Notably—and in line with its rights-based purposes—the report deploys United Nations (UN)-generated definitions—from the WHO for sexual health and from the Sustainable Development Agenda for reproductive health—as follows:

Components of Sexual Health

The report adopts the definition contained in the Sustainable Development Agenda: 'A state of physical, emotional, mental and social well-being in relation to sexuality; it is not merely the absence of disease, dysfunction or infirmity. Sexual health requires a positive and respectful approach to sexuality and sexual relationships, as well as the possibility of having pleasurable and safe sexual experiences, free of coercion, discrimination and violence.'[46]

The implications that follow from this definition are adopted from the UN Population Fund[47]—that fully realized sexual health for all would entail all people having access to:

- Counselling and care related to sexuality, sexual identity and sexual relationships
- Services for the prevention and management of sexually transmitted infections including HIV/AIDS, and other diseases of the genitourinary system
- Psychosexual counselling and treatment for sexual dysfunction and disorders
- Prevention and management of cancers of the reproductive system.

Components of Reproductive Health

'Reproductive health is a state of complete physical, mental and social well-being and not merely the absence of disease or infirmity, in all matters relating to the reproductive system and to its functions and processes.'[48]

Again, the social and medical requisites which follow from the encompass-ing definition are drawn from a variety of UN sources (with the exception of infertility)—that is, that reproductive health implies that all people are able to:

- receive accurate information about the reproductive system and the services needed to maintain reproductive health
- manage menstruation in a hygienic way, in privacy, and with dignity
- access multisectoral services to prevent and respond to intimate part-ner violence and other forms of gender-based violence
- access safe, effective, affordable and acceptable methods of contra-ception of their choice
- access appropriate health-care services to ensure safe and healthy pregnancy and childbirth, and healthy infants
- access safe abortion services, including post-abortion care
- access services for prevention, management and treatment of infertility.

Sexual Rights

Sexual rights are human rights and include the rights of all persons, free of discrimination, coercion and violence, to:

- achieve the highest attainable standard of sexual health, including access to sexual and reproductive health services
- seek, receive and impart information related to sexuality
- receive comprehensive, evidence-based sexuality education
- have their bodily integrity respected
- choose their sexual partner
- decide whether to be sexually active or not
- engage in consensual sexual relations
- choose whether, when and whom to marry
- enter into marriage with free and full consent and with equality between spouses in and at the dissolution of marriage
- pursue a satisfying, safe and pleasurable sexual life, free from stigma and discrimination
- make free, informed and voluntary decisions on their sexuality, sex-ual orientation and gender identity.

Reproductive Rights

Reproductive rights rest on the recognition of the human rights of all couples and individuals to decide freely and responsibly the number, spacing and timing of their children, to have the information and means to do so, and the right to attain the highest standard of reproductive health. They also include:

- the right to make decisions concerning reproduction free of discrimination, coercion and violence
- the right to privacy, confidentiality, respect and informed consent
- the right to mutually respectful and equitable gender relations.

The report does not sharply demarcate the components of SRH which are uncontroversial (such as ensuring safe and healthy pregnancy and childbirth, and healthy infants) from SRH as rights, as the inclusion of access to safe abortion and an acceptance of a range of sexual identities and relationships within the 'components' sub-sections clearly indicate; and these are consolidated and detailed under the 'rights' sub-sections.

Sexual and Reproductive Health as Rights

Sexual and reproductive health encompasses considerably more than merely bodies in space and time: it concerns the full expression of personhood, in all of its richness and complexity. What counts as 'relational' in sexual and reproductive health cannot be confined to either intimate and familial relations or lego-political spheres. Matters of identity, choice, control, access, freedom, individual and shared values and beliefs are inescapably bound up with biological imperatives and medical needs, and as we reviewed in Chap. 2, the construction of gender and gender roles is powerfully formative of both individual experience and the social context of sexual and reproductive health.

What is true about all other forms of human rights also applies to sexual and reproductive rights: neither widespread, lived expectation nor their enshrinement in law can lift them entirely above forms of controversy and contention. Asserting a *human* right—universal and inalienable—to the specifics of the Guttmacher-Lancet Commission and similar pronouncements is of course an assignment of values which in themselves cannot dissolve the entrenched customs, beliefs and values that run contrary to them. At the same time, however, controversies about SRH provisions as rights cannot be reduced to the 'universalism versus cultural particulars' argument which features as a mainstay of the human rights literature. This is in part because the practical entanglements of health and non-health human rights with respect to all matters relating to subsistence, life-threatening and debilitating conditions and decent living conditions make rights-based approaches to health less starkly challenging and open the way for incremental gains, at least in terms of normative acceptance if not legal codification. More fundamentally, there cannot be either normative or legal incorporation of human rights in any polity abstracted from its cultural values; it is a 'fact that culture plays a fundamental role in determining the content of human rights, making regional and local variations possible (often necessary) in the context of their implementation, adjudication, and enforcement.'[49] Where sub-Saharan Africa is concerned,

> African regional human rights instruments show a clear commitment towards mirroring the specificity of idiosyncratic African traditional characterisation of social life, which influences all its components, including the perception and structure of human rights ... Such an approach clearly recalls the conception of moderate cultural relativism, in upholding the basic core of universal rights but, at the same time, promoting and putting into practice the variations which are necessary to preserve the specific regional values.[50]

The reservations lodged by states (including African ones) to positive human rights covenants might best be viewed in this light; and similarly, the gaps in the range of SRH subjects covered by the AWP.

The journey from reproductive health as a stand-alone health matter detached from sexual rights to conceptions where the two are viewed as necessarily joined has been a long one,[51] a particularly complex and fascinating facet of the progress of human rights worldwide, at points where personal identity, self-determination, human intimacy and well-being are configured and expressed within the traditions that shape gender roles, norms and legal frameworks. The long march of human rights has over the course of more than 70 years become central not only for the protection of vulnerable individuals and groups but also for global health as we now appreciate that conception. Sexual and reproductive health rights play out over both the smallest and largest scales, in globally diverse socio-cultural settings. In addition to normative resistances, there is the more enduring tension between what is recognized as a human right and as a conditional citizen entitlement. But the principal blockages to the full attainment of sexual and reproductive health for all are not essentially legal or philosophical principles, but instead arise from the myriad difficulties of turning high principles into actionable and sustainable policy, in circumstances which, in sub-Saharan Africa, are often not at all propitious.

NOTES

1. Alison Bisset (ed), *Blackstone's International Human Rights Documents* (Oxford: Oxford University Press, 2016); and, for example, with respect to UK law: Robert G. Lee (ed), *Blackstone's Statutes on Public Law & Human rights 2017–2018* (Oxford: Oxford University Press, 2017).
2. Report of the International Commission on Intervention and State Sovereignty (2001), available at: http://responsibilitytoprotect.org/ICISS%20Report-1.pdf
3. G.A. res. 217(III)A. The obvious gender bias in this article continues to attract considerable criticism. Charlesworth, H., C. Chinkin, and S. Wright. 'Feminist Approaches to International Law,' *American Journal of International Law* 85, no. 4(1991): 613–45, Chinkin, C. (1998) International Law and Human Rights, ed. T. Evans. Manchester, Manchester University Press, pp. 105–29, Robinson, F. (1998) The limits of a rights-based approach to international ethics, ed. T. Evans. Manchester, Manchester University Press, pp. 58–76.
4. P. Kandela, 'Medical Journals and Human rights,' *The Lancet*, Vol. 352, Supplement 2 (October 1998), pp. s7–s11.
5. R. Smith, H. Hiatt and D. Bertwick, *British Medical Journal* (Clinical Research), 23 Vol. 318 (7178), January 1999, pp. 248–51.
6. Plant, R. (1989) *Can there be a right to health care?* Southampton, Institute of Health Policy Studies, p. 16.
7. Beauchamp, T. L. (1991) The Right to Health Care in a Capitalist Democracy, ed. T. J. Bole, and W. B. Bondeson. London, Klewer, pp. 53–81, Cranston, M. "Are There Any Human rights?" *Daedalus* 112, no. 4(1983): 1–18, Cranston, M. *What Are Human rights?* London: Bodley Head, 1973, Hall, M. A. "The Scope and Limits of Public Health Law." *Perspectives in Biology and Medicine* 46, no. 3(2003): 199–208, Plant, R. (1989) *Can there be a right to health care?* Southampton, Institute of Health Policy Studies, p. 16.
8. Plant, R. (1989) *Can there be a right to health care?* Southampton, Institute of Health Policy Studies, p. 16.
9. Jones, C. *Global Justice: Defending Cosmopolitanism* (Oxford: Oxford University Press, 2000).

10. J. J. Tilley, 'Cultural Relativism,' *Human rights Quarterly* 22(2) (2000), pp. 501–47.
11. Henry Shue, *Basic Rights: Subsistence, Affluence, and US Foreign Policy.* 2nd ed. (Princeton, New Jersey: Princeton University Press, 1996).
12. Ibid.
13. R. Plant, *Can there be a right to health care?* Southampton, Institute of Health Policy Studies, (1989), p. 16.
14. Henry Shue, *op cit.*
15. UN Doc. E/C.12/1992/2, p. 83, cited in David Beetham, 'What Future for Economic and Social Rights?' *Political Studies,* Vol. XLIII, Special Issue (1995), p. 41.
16. Nana Poku and Jesper Sunderwall, 'Political responsibility and global health,' *Third World Quarterly*, 04 March 2018, Vol. 39(3), pp. 471–486.
17. Thomas Risse, Stephen C. Ropp and Kethryn Sykkink (eds), *The Power of Human Rights: International Norms and Domestic Change* (Cambridge: Cambridge University Press, 1995); Alexander Betts and Phil Orchard (eds), *Implementation and World Politics: How International Norms Change Practice* (Oxford: Oxford University Press, 2014). See also: David Fidler, 'The globalization of public health: the first 100 years of international health diplomacy,' *Bulletin of the World Health Organization* Vol. 79, Issue 9, pp. 842–849; See also the special edition of *Health and Policy* on Health and Foreign Policy, in Vol. 85, Issue 3, March 2007.
18. International Coalition for the Responsibility to Protect, available at: http://responsibilitytoprotect.org
19. Millennium Development Goals 3–6: promote gender equality and empower women; reduce child mortality; improve maternal health; and combat HIV/AIDS, malaria and other diseases.
20. Nana Poku and Jim Whitman, 'The Millennium Development Goals and Development after 2015,' in Nana Poku and Jim Whitman (eds), *The Millennium Development Goals: Challenges, Prospects and Opportunities* (Abingdon: Routledge, 2014), p. 183.
21. Jennifer Brower and Peter Chalk, *The global threat of new and reemerging infectious diseases: reconciling US national security and public health policy* (Santa Monica: Rand Corporation, 2003).
22. Ellen 'T Hoen, 'TRIPS, pharmaceutical patents, and access to essential medicines: A long way from Seattle to Doha,' *Chicago Journal of International Law*, Spring 2002, Vol. 3(1), p. 31.
23. The World Bank, http://www.worldbank.org/en/topic/universalhealthcoverage
24. http://www.achpr.org/files/instruments/women-protocol/achpr_instr_proto_women_eng.pdf

25. The United Nations Millennium Declaration, available at: https://www. un.org/millennium/declaration/ares552e.htm; The Universal Declaration of Human rights, available at: https://www.un.org/en/ universal-declaration-human-rights/index.html

26. Christopher A. Tait et al., 'Can the health effects of widely-held societal norms be evaluated? An analysis of the United Nations convention on the elimination of all forms of discrimination against women (UN-CEDAW),' *BMC Public Health* (2019), 19: 279. https://doi.org/10.1186/ s12889-019-6607-6

27. A. Palmer et al., 'Does ratification of human-rights treaties have effects on population health?' *Lancet* (June 1992), doi: https://doi.org/10.1016/ S0140-6736(09)60231-2

28. Jody Heymann et al., 'Constitutional rights to health, public health and medical care: The status of health protections in 191 countries,' *Global Public Health*, 8: 6 (2013), p. 651.

29. See *UHC2030*, at uhc2030.org

30. Ana Ayala and Benjamin Mason Meier, 'Implications of food and nutrition insecurity: A human rights approach to the health,' *Public Health Reviews*, Vol. 38 (10), (2017).

31. 'Everyone has the right of access to preventive health care and the right to benefit from medical treatment under the conditions established by national laws and practices. A high level of human health protection shall be ensured in the definition and implementation of all Union policies and activities.' Charter of Fundamental Rights of the European Union, available at: http://www.europarl.europa.eu/charter/pdf/text_en.pdf

32. Tamara K. Hervey, 'We Don't See a Connection: The "Right to Health" in the EU Charter and European Social Charter,' in Gráinne de Búrca, Bruno de Witte, and Larissa Ogertschnig (eds), *Social Rights in Europe* (Oxford: Oxford University Press, 2005), p. 325.

33. Pavlos Eleftheriadis, 'A Right to Health Care,' *The Journal of Law, Medicine and Ethics* 40(2) (2012), pp. 268–85.

34. Ryder Mckeown, 'Norm Regress and the Slow Death of the Torture Norm,' *International Relations*, Vol. 23, 1 (March 2009), pp. 5–25.

35. Alicia Ely Yamin, 'Will We Take Suffering Seriously? Reflections on What Applying a Human rights Framework to Health Means and Why We Should Care,' *Health and Human Rights* 10(1), (2008), p. 50.

36. L. B. Pizzarossa and K. Perehudoff, 'Global Survey of National Constitutions: Mapping Constitutional Commitments to Sexual and Reproductive Health and Rights,' *Health and Human Rights*, 19(2) (2017), pp. 279–293.

37. Jane Cottingham et al., 'Using human rights for sexual and reproductive health: Improving legal and regulatory frameworks,' *Bulletin of the World Health Organization*, 88(7) (2010), pp. 551–5.

38. For example, see: M. Heywood, 'South Africa's Treatment Action Campaign: Combining law and social mobilization to realize the right to health,' *Journal of Human Rights Practice* 1 (2009), pp. 14–36.

39. George J. Annas, 'The Right to Health and the Nevirapine Case in South Africa,' *New England Journal of Medicine* 348 (2003), p. 751.

40. Alicia Ely Yamin, 'Promoting Equity in Health: What Role for Courts?' *Health and Human Rights*, 16(2) (December 2014), p. 2; and in the same edition, L. Colleen Flood and Aeyal Gross, 'Litigating the Right to Health: What Can We Learn from a Comparative Law and Health Care Systems Approach?' pp. 62–72.

    See also: Ebenezer Durojaye (ed), *Litigating the Right to Health in Africa: Challenges and Prospects* (Farnham: Ashgate, 2015); Jonathan Berger, 'Litigating for Social Justice in Post-Apartheid South Africa: A Focus on Health and Education,' in Varun Gauri and Daniel M. Binks (eds), *Courting Social Justice: Judicial Enforcement of Social and Economic Rights in the Developing World* (Cambridge: Cambridge University Press, 2009), pp. 38–99; Marius Pieterse, 'Health, Social Movements, and Rights-based Litigation in South Africa,' *Journal of Law and Society*, Vol. 35, No. 3 (September 2008), pp. 364–88; and 'The Law, the Courts, and Sexual and Reproductive Rights.' *Reproductive Health Matters*, vol. 22, no. 44, (2014), p. 222.

41. Keith Syrett, 'Evolving the Right to Health: Rethinking the Normative Response to Problems of Judicialization,' *Health and Human rights* 20(1), June 2018, pp. 121–32; Emmanuel Kolawole Oke, 'Incorporating a right to health perspective into the resolution of patent law disputes,' *Health and Human rights* Vol. 15, No. 2 (December 2013), pp. 97–109.

42. Joel E. Cohen, *How Many People Can the Earth Support?* (New York: Norton, 1996).

43. Steven Epstein and Laura Mamo, 'The proliferation of sexual health: Diverse social problems and the legitimation of sexuality,' *Social Science and Medicine* 18 (2017), pp. 180–83.

44. Ibid., p. 187.

45. Ann M. Starrs, et al., 'Accelerate progress—sexual and reproductive health and rights for all: report of the Guttmacher-*Lancet* Commission,' *The Lancet* 391 (2018), pp. 2642–92.

46. WHO, *Sexual health and its linkages to reproductive health: an operational approach* (Geneva: World Health Organization, 2017).

47. UN Population Fund, Population Council, 'Planning and implementing an essential package of sexual and reproductive health services'

(2011), available at: http://www.unfpa.org/resources/planning-and-mplementing-essential-package-sexual-and-reproductive-health-services

48. United Nations, 'Transforming our world: the 2030 agenda for sustainable development,' A/RES/70/1. New York, NY: United Nations, 2015.
49. Federico Lenzerini, *The Culturalization of Human rights Law* (Oxford: Oxford University Press, 2014), p. 216.
50. Ibid., p. 58.
51. Carmen Barroso, 'From reproductive to sexual rights,' in Peter Aggleton and Richard Parker (eds), *Routledge Encyclopedia of Sexuality, Health and Rights* (Abingdon: Routledge, 2010), pp. 379–88.

CHAPTER 4

Sexual and Reproductive Health in Sub-Saharan Africa: Normative Developments, Contexts and Issues

Abstract This chapter concerns the normative dimensions of sexual and reproductive health (SRH) as applied to sub-Saharan contexts and issues. The positive impacts of growing international consensus around SRH are contrasted with both the normative and practical limitations. The conditioning sub-Saharan contexts include demography; gender; HIV and other SRH-related disease burdens; and health systems and health systems funding. The highly diverse normative landscape of sub-Saharan Africa is illustrated by attitudes towards and provision of contraception and abortion.

Keywords Demography • HIV • Health systems • Contraception • Abortion

The conditions which determine and shape sexual and reproductive health (SRH) throughout the world cannot be restricted to a single realm, level of human interaction, lego-political arena or prevailing social norm. The range of vulnerabilities is too wide and the lines of causation creating and/or sustaining them are too complex for all-embracing abstractions. We have a considerable array of worrying statistics on SRH, but facts don't speak for themselves, and the values attached to matters sexual and reproductive are powerful. This is not to suggest that we are helpless in the face

© The Author(s), under exclusive license to Springer Nature Singapore Pte Ltd. 2020
N. K. Poku, *Sexual and Reproductive Health and Rights in Sub-Saharan Africa*, Global Research in Gender, Sexuality and Health, https://doi.org/10.1007/978-981-15-8502-9_4

of human complexity but that how we conceive SRH as an 'issue' has a powerful bearing on our sense of human consequences, and on our ability and willingness as well as our practical capacity to act. The history of the evolving response to the AIDS pandemic over three decades illustrates this.[1]

The promotion of SRH as a human right is effectively an effort to supplant forms and degrees of issue relegation, selective blindness and restricted entitlement. It is a powerful concept because it is wholly inclusive; because it brings SRH within both legal and political realms, nationally and internationally; and because it immediately invokes obligations. But broad international commitments notwithstanding, SRH as a human right struggles to gain traction in the same ways as other positive human rights—and for many the same reasons. Sub-Saharan African states are by no means unique in their reluctance to recognize sexual and reproductive health as human rights beyond the formalities of the principal international covenants. Yet even outside considerations of SRH as a human right, advances in SRH as foundations for sustainable development in Africa have not only found consensus but have also been formalized.

Over more than two decades, focused and sustained development initiatives—first, the Millennium Development Goals (MDGs) and currently, though to a lesser degree, the Sustainable Development Goals (SDGs)—have given high priority to health, with a particular emphasis on gender as a key component of propelling and sustaining development more generally.[2] (As briefly outlined in Chap. 2, five of the eight Millennium Development Goals were dedicated either to SRH issues or to gender equality.) The confluence of the goal- and target-specific MDGs with the weight of evidence placing gender equality and SRH at the centre of human development has led to some remarkable and detailed African initiatives. Through a range of international covenants and especially through the declarations of the African Union (AU), African states have firmly committed themselves to affirming the centrality of the key relational element in sexual and reproductive health—gender equality. The AU's visionary declaration, *Africa 2063: The Future We Want*[3] calls for 'an entrenched and flourishing culture of human rights [and] gender equality,' for the elimination of 'all forms of gender-based violence and discrimination' and asserts that 'Africa must provide an enabling environment for its women, children and young people to flourish and reach their full potential.'

From an explicit SRH perspective, *Africa 2063* appears disappointing since aside from foreseeing the end of female genital mutilation and child marriages, 'health' is included only as a long-range goal, alongside such matters as world-class infrastructure—and sexual and reproductive health not at all. But *Africa 2063* is a strategic vision for development writ large, not a roadmap; it is a consolidation of continent-wide ambition and strategic thinking. The gradual movement of gender equality and SRH to the forefront of development received its earliest, most direct and powerful expression at the Fifth International Conference on Population and Development (ICPD) in 1994, when 179 governments signed on to the ICPD Programme of Action. It was a radical conceptual departure from how world population had been conceived and how 'development' had been promoted and practised in previous decades. As articulated by the United Nations Population Fund (UNFPA) at the 20-year mark, '[T]he ICPD Programme of Action marked a fundamental shift in global thinking on population and development issues. It moved away from a focus on reaching specific demographic targets to a focus on the needs, aspirations and rights of individual women and men. The Programme of Action asserted that everyone counts, that the true focus of development policy must be the improvement of individual lives and the measure of progress should be the extent to which we address inequalities.'[4]

A year after the fifth ICPD, the fourth UN Conference on Women was held in Beijing (the first having taken place in 1975, followed by five-yearly reviews).[5]

Although the Conferences and their follow-ups had as their remit gender equality and the empowerment of women rather than women's health or SRH in particular, they gained from and added to the momentum which is even now helping to maintain both gender and SRH as a sine qua non of development.

On the 20th anniversary of ICPD 1994, the *ICPD Beyond 2014 Review* produced a report which affirmed an international agenda, setting out in explicit terms the primacy of sexual and reproductive health, grounded in gender equality:

Priority actions by governments, development partners, civil society, private sector and the international community include the following:

- Reaffirm that sexual and reproductive rights are universal human rights, meaning that they are existing rights in national and international human rights instruments to which every individual is entitled by virtue of being a human being, irrespective of age, sex, race and ethnicity, religion, language, physical or intellectual disability, health status (including HIV/AIDS), gender identity, sexual orientation, intersex or transgender status, marital status or any other status, and that their exercise is essential for the enjoyment of all other human rights and for achieving social justice and sustainable development.

- Bring laws and regulations that criminalize or otherwise impinge on sexual and reproductive rights into accord with international human rights obligations and laws, including those that restrict access, overall or to particular groups, to comprehensive sexuality education and information, that criminalize consensual same-sex relations or sex work, or that deny specific services including contraception and safe abortion services, among others.

- Promote policies that enable the full exercise of sexual and reproductive rights, embracing the right to a safe and full sex life, as well as the right to take free, informed, voluntary and responsible decisions on sexuality and reproduction, without coercion, discrimination or violence, and that guarantee the right to information and the means necessary for attaining the highest standards of sexual health and reproductive health.

- Develop and fully implement policies and special initiatives—and dedicate sufficient resources—to ensure universal access to the full range of sexual and reproductive health services, information and education, regardless of individuals' capacity to pay service fees and other costs, giving priority attention to access for those who are disadvantaged and marginalized (e.g., location of facilities and allocation of outreach workers, transport, alternatives to facility-based services, special programmes to reach the most vulnerable including, such as, adolescent girls living in poverty or indigenous communities living in remote rural areas).

- Take all necessary legal, policy, programming, budgeting, judicial or any other measures at national, sub-national and community level to end all forms of gender-based violence and harmful practices such as early and forced marriage, female genital mutilation, among others, including in conflict and humanitarian settings.

- Ensure that customary or religious laws and practices do not infringe on people's rights, particularly women's rights, maintaining dialogue with traditional, faith-based and community leaders and other influential persons to promote interpretations of these laws in conformity with international human rights law.[6]

Perhaps the most notable achievement in placing SRH and gender equality as a potentially actionable agenda throughout sub-Saharan Africa (SSA) was the sequence of AU agreements beginning with the Continental Policy Framework on Sexual and Reproductive Health and Rights, 2005.[7] This was followed by the Maputo Plan of Action, 2007–10 (subsequently extended to 2015) and the Maputo Plan of Action, 2016–30.[8] The last of these contains a detailed list of Strategic Focus and Priority Interventions 2016–30 as well as aggregate outline costings.

The Limits of SRHR Normative Congruence

The formal AU commitments to SRH demonstrate an encouraging degree of congruence with broader international agreements, particularly the ICPD and its successive reviews. But the AU does not directly engage sexual health except as an integral component of reproductive health; and despite most African countries' accession in other forums to the concept of sexual and reproductive health rights, the language adopted by the AU reveals the political sensitivity of doing so in ways that might entail controversial political or legal obligations—hence the carefully phrased title of the AU Continental Policy Framework, on 'sexual and reproductive health *and* rights.' There is much about the Maputo agreements to commend,[9] and it is certainly an advance to have closely inter-related health and social issues framed together. These include contraceptive use, maternal and child health, sexually transmitted diseases (STDs), family planning, population pressures, abortion, teenage pregnancy, gender equality, education, marriage and sexual and reproductive decisions. But the importance of sexual health extends well beyond its reproductive implications and outcomes, with sexual identity and same-sex relationships a particularly sensitive area. Again, these sensitivities are not unique to African constituencies, but the demographic profile together with SRH statistical indicators for sub-Saharan Africa as a whole gives them considerable salience. And even within the category of reproductive health, the agenda with respect to abortion in the latest Maputo Plan of Action is on reducing the number of unsafe abortions; and the sole mention of providing access to safe abortions is that it should be made ' in accordance with national laws and policies.' Increasing normative congruence at international and continental levels does serve the purpose of bringing SRH issues fully into the political and policy-making spheres, but it does not necessarily make them readily actionable—and may indeed provoke national and local backlashes. Hence the caution of political leaders and governments.

Within the wider sphere of development, the agenda of the SDGs is a very considerable expansion of the highly focused MDGs. The SDGs are of unprecedented proportions, with many of its largest issue areas matters of some urgency requiring both sustained political commitment and considerable levels of funding. It is already clear that even the global fight against HIV and AIDS, let alone SRH more generally, will have to compete with the full panoply of human development aspirations, including action on climate change, marine conservation, urbanization initiatives and sustainable economic growth. However well-integrated the plan is in prospect, the programmatic difficulties entailed in 17 goals and 169 targets, spread across nearly every important aspect of planetary sustainability and human equity, are likely to create hard choices, difficult decisions about prioritization, competition for resources and the familiar difficulties of ensuring that commitments are honoured and sustained. The greatly reduced standing of SRH in the SDGs compared to the MDGs is already visible in the levelling off of funding for the AIDS pandemic—to some degree triggered by the financial crash of 2008, but also by the loss of its profile as a uniquely urgent global issue in the face of others, around which normative expectation at popular, donor and government levels has begun to coalesce.

The emergence, articulation, promulgation and growth of normative expectation in any field is never sufficient on its own for practical purposes, but it does serve the vital role of helping to make conditions—whether dire circumstances, public hazards, environmental harms or human vulnerabilities, into matters of public and political concern—that is, into issues. As with the history of human rights, the worth of the necessary-but-insufficient normative impetus is easy to under-estimate when set against the scale of preventable harms and the time usually required to move from nominal agreements to policy planning and implementation.

The limiting and conditioning factors that shape the prospects for giving practical expression to the normative progress towards gender equality and towards sexual and reproductive health can be grouped under three themes. The first is high-level political. Although the Sustainable Development Goals, the Maputo Plan of Action and *Africa 2063* are unprecedented commitments, these and other international resolutions must find the largest part of their practical expression through countries that have committed to them. This theme gives rise to four kinds of difficulty. The first is the familiar problem of securing sufficient (and sufficiently enduring) commitment from states (including, but not limited to, finance) to ensure that their promises are fulfilled. The second is the problem of competing interests and difficult choices, even within the compass of acknowledged rights or obligations. Third, what makes these and similar commitments so challenging isn't only the scope of the issues, but that they require sustained political commitment and considerable levels of funding, often against the volatilities of the international political economy and the vagaries of election cycles. The failure to fully enact the succession of international climate change agreements continues to display all three of those features. Fourth, it requires very skilful leadership to determine and coordinate holistic versus country- and issue-specific initiatives, particularly where considerable amounts of donor funds are necessary.

The second theme is conceptual—that is, how we conceive a condition or an issue to be addressed as a matter of public health policy. Of course, there are health policy emergencies which vault over such considerations—the 2014–15 Ebola outbreak in West Africa, for example—but in general, the sexual and reproductive health of populations can take the form of relatively discrete, single issues (accessible and affordable provision of SRH clinics; the availability of legal, safe abortions); as large issues such as the availability of safe and reliable contraceptives, which can both arise from and encompass socio-cultural and national-developmental priorities as well as more direct, large-scale health considerations[10]; and in the case of HIV and AIDS, although the scale, impacts and causal dynamics largely have their origin in the realm of sexual health, it has over time not only become a very large cluster of issues (encompassing but extending beyond SRH) but also a matter that has for decades conditioned practically every other aspect of health policy planning and financing in many SSA countries. We cannot reasonably choose to plan and act as though SRH is a single issue, and setting priorities and demarcating areas of focus in order to maximize as broad a range of benefits as possible is an act of ordering that, at times, can result in the relegation or exclusion of others.

The third theme is the relationship between the personal and the political—that is, the links between private behaviours and very large public outcomes. How societies reconcile the demands and tensions between freedom and order is at the heart of political philosophy and also of human rights—and sexual and reproductive matters offer countless points of friction in this regard, through laws, social norms and the cultural particulars which frame the boundaries of both acceptable behaviours and acceptable public policy. But the difficulties of addressing SRH in sub-Saharan Africa extend beyond certain socio-cultural fixtures and taboos. This is because the individual and relational sources of deleterious, large-scale SRH issues often frustrate our perceptions of causal relations, rational self-interest and calculable risk aversion—particularly when our purposes are preventive rather than curative. In addition, the myriad causal and formative conditions that shape sexual behaviours and reproductive outcomes are themselves complex phenomena, including poverty, migration,[11] rapid urbanization[12] and gender inequalities[13]—and the nature and degree to which they act as SRH determinants is sometimes counterintuitive. For example:

> Despite the popular and rhetorical attention that has been given to the role that poverty plays as an underlying cause of HIV in SSA, the cumulative evidence suggests that there is a need for a much more nuanced understanding of the interaction between poverty and HIV, especially in the context of low- and middle-income countries. The social epidemiology of HIV belies simplistic assumptions that negative health outcomes will always disproportionately accrue to the poor.[14]

Throughout the world, social and political sensitivities about SRH as rights and about addressing certain issues, particularly those arising from gender values, including sexual identities and behaviours (but also procreative matters, especially contraception and abortion) arise from a variety of sources and take many forms. What generates an impression of sub-Saharan African exceptionalism over sexual and reproductive rights is that the conditions are so burdensome and the human consequences so great. It is to these that we now turn.

Sexual and Reproductive Health in Sub-Saharan Africa: Contexts and Issues

Contexts

Demography
The demography of Africa critically shapes the prospects for promoting and securing a healthy future for its peoples, in line with Goal 5 of the SDGs and the broader aspirations of *Africa 2063: The Future We Want.*

That is because Africa has a very young age profile, with about two-fifths of its population in the 0–14 age bracket (approximately 486 million children) and nearly one-fifth (19 per cent) in the 15–24 age bracket (approximately 230 million young people). According to the World Bank, 'Of the world's top ten countries with the youngest populations, eight are in sub-Sahara Africa. By 2050, the region will be home to all 10.'[15]

Decades of calls for population control based on demographic projections and with a view towards development (and increasingly, planetary sustainability) have had a mixed and, at times, controversial history.[16] Whether there is a necessary connection and a one-way dynamic between a drop in fertility rates and the history of industrial/economic development outside of Africa and the extent to which other factors were in play and significantly formative, it remains the case that sustained changes in fertility rates bring about 'demographic transitions' of various kinds, with all of their concomitant policy-making challenges. (Witness the ageing 'baby boomer' populations in the West.) However, there is strong consensus in international forums and organizations, including the African Union, that the most basic forms of stability and sustainability are imperilled by high fertility rates—here expressed in a report by the Organisation for Economic Co-operation and Development (OECD):

> Although population growth has decelerated in most countries, the world's population is still growing at a high rate. Without a significant and rapid drop in fertility rates it could reach 16 billion by 2100, according to the latest projections of the United Nations Population Division. Population growth, coupled with higher consumption, raises the stakes in our efforts to reduce poverty, create employment, provide food, water and energy security, while safeguarding the natural environment.

There immediately follows the call for universal access to SRH:

> To promote sustainable development pathways, developing countries and their partners will need to ensure: i) universal access to sexual and reproductive health care and family planning; ii) investment in education with a particular focus on gender parity; iii) empowerment of women; and iv) systematic integration of population projections in development strategies and policies.[17]

It is true that 'demography is not destiny'; that fertility rates vary considerably within SSA; and that so long as the highest fertility rates decrease at a sufficient rate, there can be considerable advantages to the youth bulge in developing parts of the world, SSA not least.[18] But at the largest scales, including but not limited to SSA, the need for accessible, high-quality SRH services is clearly fundamental.

That need is no less pressing as a matter for the health and well-being of individuals, families and communities—and filling unmet contraceptive needs would deliver benefits at both the most fundamental as well as the highest scales. For example, '[i]ncreasing contraceptive prevalence has already reduced adolescent fertility by 6.8 per cent in Latin America and 4.1 per cent in sub-Saharan Africa. Meeting the total demand for contraceptives of unmarried adolescents would lead to an additional decrease in fertility of 8.9 per cent and 17.4 per cent respectively.'[19]

For decades to come, the youthful populations of SSA countries will confront the complex physical, psychological, emotional and social changes that take place during adolescence—in numbers that would be difficult to cater for even in the best circumstances. This has both immediate and long-term implications for both individuals and their societies—not least as the onset of puberty ushers in the initiation of sexual activity, and subsequent exposure to the risk of unwanted pregnancy and sexually transmitted infection (STIs), including HIV. Awareness of sexual orientation also emerges during this period, as do the onset of mental health disorders. Increased risk-taking and a heightened sensitivity to peers may lead to risky behaviours.

HIV and SRH-Related Disease Burdens
The behavioural/preventive facets of reproductive health are of course not limited to the risk of unwanted pregnancies or to larger national and/or international demographic concerns. Biologically and medically, behaviourally induced sexual and reproductive health vulnerabilities often appear together, with preventable harms in sexual health often having serious impacts on reproductive health, as is the case with mother-to-child transmission of HIV. And although globally, approximately 1.6 per cent of all maternal deaths are estimated to be AIDS-related, in sub-Saharan Africa that figure is 2 per cent; and in 2015 there were five countries where the figures are estimated to be 10 per cent or more: South Africa (32 per cent), Swaziland (19 per cent), Botswana (18 per cent), Lesotho (13 per cent) and Mozambique (11 per cent).[20]

To this must be added the reproductive risks that accompany the range of STIs currently at epidemic levels:

Sexually transmitted infections (STIs) are among the most common acute conditions worldwide. WHO estimated in 2012 that there were 357·4 million new global cases of four common curable STIs: chlamydia (130·9 million cases), gonorrhoea (78·3 million cases), syphilis (5·6 million cases), and trichomoniasis (142·6 million cases). Additionally, there are alarming increases in antimicrobial resistance in [some strains.] Although most STIs are not usually fatal, they result in a substantial burden of disease. The complications of curable STIs include pelvic inflammatory disease, ectopic pregnancy, infertility, chronic pelvic pain, seronegative arthropathy, and neurological and cardiovascular diseases. STIs in pregnancy can cause fetal or neonatal death, premature delivery, and neonatal encephalitis, eye infections, and pneumonia. STIs can also increase the infectiousness of and susceptibility to HIV. Despite these complications, STIs remain a neglected field for clinical and public health practice and for research.[21]

Once HIV and AIDS had been acknowledged as a public health emergency, the urgent and continuing need to increase and make more effective HIV prevention also necessitated a powerful and sustained focus on sexual and reproductive health, but for historical reasons, in some sub-Saharan African countries the programmatic tasks of linking the two were a challenge:

[A]t the time of the emergence of HIV in sub-Saharan Africa, many family planning programs were still quite new, and in their quest to be successful, focused on marital sex. As such, the contemporaneous HIV programs that targeted sex workers could not operate through the existing structures related to family planning. Donors also knew that African governments had been resistant to family planning, and so did not want to associate HIV with such a controversial topic. Bureaucratic structuring also separated family planning from HIV: ministries of health initially placed HIV with sexually transmitted infections, rather than with maternal health and family planning. In addition, family planning programs generally did not promote condoms as a means of contraception.[22]

Further, 'the positive association between population policy adoption and HIV outcomes may reflect an impact of policy feedback in that governments experienced with adopting policy in the realm of the intimate were more likely to engage in other intimate interventions.'[23]

Despite the unprecedented global response to the AIDS pandemic and the remarkably diverse rates of prevalence throughout SSA—from less than 1 per cent in Madagascar and Somalia to more than 20 per cent in

Botswana, Lesotho and Swaziland—the principal statistical indicators across the region remain stark. The gains made against the disease are considerable: according to the Joint United Nations Programme on HIV and AIDS (UNAIDS), roughly half of the people living with HIV (approximately 23 million) are now accessing antiretroviral therapy, for whom the disease is now chronic, rather than life-threatening. But even as the enrolment of people carrying the HIV virus onto ART continues, ground is being lost to new infections—approximately two million per year; and it has been estimated by UNAIDS that more than eight million people do not know they are living with HIV.

There is no viable substitute for re-energizing, funding and supporting culturally attuned, locally staffed HIV advocacy and prevention programmes, especially in resource-poor settings. The evidence that such interventions are effective remains compelling; and although the cost implications are not negligible, the medium to long-term outcomes must be regarded not as complementary, but as integral to biomedical interventions. The success of the antiretroviral drugs upscale has enabled a noticeable improvement in AIDS-related morbidity and mortality in the recent years, yet the underlying dynamics of the epidemic remain determined by the rate at which new infections are taking place in relation to the number of AIDS deaths. While the rate of new HIV infections is stabilizing in some of the hardest hit countries, it remains far too high and the future cost of maintaining an ever-expanding pool of people reliant on daily drugs for survival is unsustainable.[24] As expressed in a World Bank Study:

> Most international resources are earmarked for treatment. The only way to stem the need for treatment and save lives is to push for serious and expansive prevention initiatives. An in-depth evaluation of the U.S. PEPFAR [President's Emergency Plan for AIDS Relief] program concludes that it reduced deaths by 5 per cent but had no effect on prevention. The recent multimillion dollar evaluation of the Global Fund noted the organization's neglect of prevention. A more modest review assessing the programs of the World Bank, Global Fund, and PEPFAR also concluded that prevention was the weak link in each institution's program. The challenge is that for every HIV/AIDS patient placed on treatment, two or three newly infected people will need treatment for life.[25]

Countries must exercise caution in continuing to focus on treatment as a 'quick fix' to end AIDS as a public health concern. HIV is a socially and culturally induced crisis and, as such, a variety of measures are needed simultaneously to appeal to different people, groups and circumstances—which is precisely what accessible, well-resourced SRH services provide.[26]

The social and cultural drivers of HIV and AIDS restore us to the point that sexual and reproductive health is concerned with persons, in all of their individuality and relational complexities, not merely bodies. Medical interventions matter, but logically, reducing the number of them has a prior claim. But as we have reviewed more generally, powerful social norms can also block outreach, screening, detection and treatment for what are now referred to as 'key populations,' so termed because the risk of acquiring HIV is 22 times higher among men who have sex with men; 22 times higher among people who inject drugs; 21 times higher for sex workers; and 12 times higher for transgender people.[27] To this list must be added prisoners and people with disabilities. Sexual identities, relationships and behaviours deemed illicit and/or made illegal remain a serious difficulty for slowing the spread of HIV and for the provision of sexual and reproductive health services for them. The fear of persecution and/or prosecution under prohibitive legal regimes results in gender and sexual minorities 'hiding' or 'hidden' populations. (In more than half of African countries, same-sex relationships are illegal,[28] but there has been progress in decriminalization, and with respect to HIV, most notably in South Africa.) The dangers extend beyond the professed boundaries of sexual identity, in part because of transactional sex; and because sexual behaviours often stray beyond the labels we attach to ourselves and others.[29]

On many reckonings, adolescents and young adults can also be regarded as a key population in the struggle against AIDS through the provision of SRH services. This is because most adolescents have little experience of navigating health systems, and they are less willing to seek services; when they do, they may find health workers have unhelpful or judgemental attitudes; and the service providers themselves can find themselves awkwardly placed between medical need, legal strictures and their own moral standards.[30] For adolescents who are often not aware of their rights, policies and laws specifying age-related restrictions and stipulating consent by parents/guardians or spouses[31] add to their fears and deter those who might otherwise seek services. At the same time, such official restrictions create complex dilemmas for providers who want to act in the best interest of their clients but who may have concerns about their own legal liability as well as the safety of their young clients.[32] More than at any other life stage, adolescent health is strongly determined by social context. Both the large, structural determinants of health (e.g., national wealth, income inequality and access to health services) and more proximate determinants such as connectedness to family and school affect health-related behaviour and outcomes during adolescence.[33]

Gender

But there is a further structural determinant to adult as well as adolescent SRH vulnerability: the disproportionate SRH risks and harms suffered by girls and young women, which is conveyed by the brute reality that, according to the WHO, in some settings up to 45 per cent of adolescent girls report that their first sexual experience was forced.[34] Added to this are many other varieties of female disempowerment: fewer educational and employment opportunities; poverty facilitating age-discordant sexual relations, transactional sex and low age of sexual debut; insufficient knowledge and/or lack of affordable access to SRH services in order for women to control their fertility; and a variety of socially validated male prerogatives which give women little room for negotiating the particulars of sexual relationships, whether in or outside marriage.

Gender inequality is at the root of nearly every sexual and reproductive harm in SSA, directly or indirectly—and the statistics bear this out, not least in respect of HIV and AIDS: according to UNAIDS, in sub-Saharan Africa, four in five new infections among adolescents aged 15–19 are in girls. Young women aged 15–24 years are twice as likely to be living with HIV than men of the same age. Similar disparities hold for STIs, as a result of the complex interplay between contextual factors that cannot be reduced to physiology: 'The difference in prevalence of STIs between men and women is especially marked in young people under the age of 25. The discrepancies [...] cannot only be explained by more efficient transmission from men to women than from women to men. The high vulnerability to STIs of young women compared to young men is the result of an interplay between psychological, sociocultural, and biological factors.'[35]

There is an extensive literature on correlations between disturbing statistical indicators for SRH and the varieties and degrees to which girls and women are variously constricted in their freedoms and options, marginalized, excluded, exploited and repressed, not only in sexual matters but also in broader social terms—and much of that research underpins international as well as African Union declarations and policy pronouncements on the centrality of gender equality. Notably, a wide range of preventive and ameliorative initiatives to address SRH morbidities and vulnerabilities extend beyond medical and health system interventions but are addressed at improving the circumstances of girls and young women.[36] But as discussed in Chap. 2, the encompassing normative tenor of societies which form the boundaries and shape the qualities of intimate relations will not usually be given to sudden change, at least by way of lego-political strictures—as is evident from the halting progress made in eliminating early and child marriages in sub-Saharan Africa (one of the targets for Goal 5 of the SDGs):

> High levels of child marriage persist throughout much of sub-Saharan Africa despite legislative efforts to prevent the practice. By 2010, 25 of the 31 countries [under study] had set a minimum legal age for marriage at 18 years or older. Guinea, Niger, Togo, Chad, the Democratic Republic of Congo, and Zimbabwe were exceptions and had legal minimums between 15 and 17 years of age. All 31 countries permit exceptions to the minimum in the case of consent from parents or religious or judicial authorities. Although these laws represent an important precedent for the protection of human rights, [it appears likely] that they are insufficient to eliminate the practice. Given the numerous exceptions to the minimum age, even rigorous enforcement of existing laws is unlikely to eliminate child marriage.[37]

Health Systems and Health Systems Funding
The scale of the need to combat HIV and AIDS throughout much of SSA over the last two decades—and certainly in the worst-affected countries—propelled a scale-up of at least some dedicated SRH services. But it also presented health policy-makers with unanticipated consequences, ethical quandaries and difficult choices over whether and how the advances in SRH services for HIV and AIDS purposes can be consolidated, extended and/or sustained at a time of steep declines in dedicated development assistance and increasing demands for a range of other health issues including but extending beyond SRH. Given the dependence of resource-poor, high HIV prevalence states in SSA, the foreign assistance trajectory is troubling in itself and for its implications:

> [The] decline in development assistance for HIV/AIDS [was] 23 per cent between 2013 and 2015. The decline is concerning for the countries in which development assistance for HIV/AIDS plays a substantial role and where the burden of HIV/AIDS remains high. This is of particular concern in sub-Saharan Africa which is home to 24.4 million people living with HIV/AIDS as of 2015, the most across regions. Spending on HIV/AIDS

in sub-Saharan Africa is financed predominantly from external sources, with Development Assistance constituting 63.9 per cent of all HIV/AIDS spending in the region in 2015.[38]

Worryingly, the reduced pattern of donor support for HIV/AIDS may impact prevention efforts:

> The uneven declines across prevalence groups suggest development assistance partners are firmer in their commitment to supporting extremely high-prevalence countries, which maintain large antiretroviral therapy (ART) programs. The prevention programs critical to slowing transmission of HIV in low- and high-prevalence countries, however, may be at risk.[39]

The legacy issues generated by the HIV/AIDS SRH scale-up include both general and country-specific calls for the integration of AIDS financing into larger national health systems budgets. Since the millennium, many high-level studies have been devoted to how best to fund the health systems of low-income countries; and more recently, on the prospects for establishing Universal Health Care (UHC) systems and on strengthened health systems sufficient for the incorporation of HIV/AIDS services.[40] But while there is evidence that 'scale-up of HIV services has produced stronger health systems and conversely, that stronger health systems were critical to the success of HIV scale-up,'[41] this is not a sufficient basis on which to plan the integration of HIV funding, but rather a reflection of the sheer scale of the ART roll-out and its associated health support services.

There are long-running debates about the pros and cons of organizing disease-specific health system responses as relatively free-standing 'vertical' programmes or in more 'horizontal' configurations,[42] but the scale and urgency of the AIDS pandemic ensured a largely vertical approach, much abetted by donor-driven agendas, largely outside of the strategic direction of African health ministries. What is at risk when funding for such programmatic and infrastructural arrangements is run down is that the issue of a transition to 'country ownership' in many cases is likely to present as a crisis because transitions of this kind need to be tailored to individual country circumstances—and that requires considerable planning and cooperation[43] in order to ensure not only that the risk to breaks in coverage is minimized but also that the transition is sustainable.[44] Countries unable to fully cover funding shortfalls through efficiencies or alternative funding sources will struggle to accommodate one or both of HIV/

AIDS-specific and more general SRH screening and treatment needs.[45] To this must be added the inefficiencies which will arise from patchy infrastructures, weak bureaucracies and the poor governance of some SSA health systems.[46]

In addition to the implications of the changing donor landscape for SSA health systems generally, there is a long-standing programmatic case for integrating HIV and AIDS services into existing SRH service provision, particularly with respect to family planning and maternal/child health. Advocacy for this dates from the IPCD 1994 conference[47] and was reinforced at the WHO/UNFPA Gilion consultation on strengthening the linkages between reproductive health and HIV/AIDS, on the reasoning that family planning and the prevention of HIV in women and children entails bridging the gaps between services for women accessing family planning, testing and counselling, or antenatal care programmes. The recommendations reveal in practical terms the ways in which sexual and reproductive health are inextricable:

- HIV counselling should be integrated into family planning services in order to address the dual risk of infection and unintended pregnancy women face in their lives.
- HIV testing and counselling should be integrated into family planning programmes, and testing and counselling programmes should provide contraceptive counselling, especially on the consistent and correct use of condoms. This will enable women who learn that they are HIV-positive to access contraception, if desired, and will help women who are uninfected to avoid HIV infection and unintended pregnancy.
- HIV testing and counselling, safer sex counselling and family planning counselling and services (including condoms) should be provided in antenatal and post-natal care settings. This will help pregnant women to avoid infection and will help to identify pregnant women with HIV, who can be offered post-partum contraceptive counselling and services for the prevention of subsequent pregnancies, if this is desired.[48]

The case is compelling, but implementation is beset by broader health system weaknesses and fixtures that require dedicated and resourced change management. So '[d]espite the long-standing global recognition of the need for the integration of basic health and SRH services with HIV services [there are] inter-related systems factors at policy and service-delivery inhibiting the delivery of integrated care. Separate policies, guidelines, ministerial directorates, under-funding of SRH, program territorialism, weak management systems, vertical training programs, lack of monitoring and evaluation systems, and ineffective referral systems [are all] critical barriers to integration. Providers therefore understandably struggle to cope with multiple health programming and service delivery requirements. The capacity of already overburdened staff to address diverse and broad client health needs also remains a concern given human resource [shortages]."[49]

In addition to the challenges of how SRH services can best be financed and configured, comprehensive sexual and reproductive health care in the countries of sub-Saharan Africa cannot entirely or even largely be reduced to physiology and medicine. That is because the deepest sources of preventable sexual and reproductive harms are human vulnerabilities rather than microbial infections—that is, they are normative and relational in origin, with gender inequality as the principal enabler, leaving so many girls and young women exposed to infection, impairment and injury. The immediate causes are numerous and pervasive, including gender-based violence with high risks of direct physical injury; unintended pregnancy; risk of HIV and other STIs; and mental health disorders.[50] Other indicators of the SRH impacts of gender inequality include the estimate that half of all births in southern Africa occur in adolescence, a million to girls younger than 16 who are four times more likely to die in pregnancy or childbirth than the 20–24–year-old cohort; resort to illegal abortions (discussed below); the declining but persistent practice of female genital mutilation, with some three million girls per year thought to be at risk; and in the worst-affected countries, adolescent girls account for more than 80 per cent of new HIV infections in their age group.[51]

The centrality of gender equality for sexual and reproductive health has been recognized for decades—it features in the 1994 ICPD Programme of Action (at 4.4(a)); and in the targets for Sustainable Development Goal 5.[52] Both of these commitments and others implicitly acknowledge that SRH cannot be wholly medicalized; that dealing with the drivers of terrible, near-systemic SRH outcomes requires a broadened conception of what counts as a medical intervention, particularly for preventive purposes; and that the conditions under which adolescents—and girls and young women especially—live and come to maturity need to inform the remit of SR clinics and health systems more generally.

As a consequence, much energy is now invested in community-based engagement and inputs for the furtherance of healthy adolescent sexuality, and one study advocates a comprehensive, 'ecological' approach, entailing every relational level:

- At the individual level, there is a need to focus on empowering adolescents including through efforts such as those that build the economic and social assets as well as the resources of adolescents.
- At the relationship level, there is a need to build relationships that support and reinforce positive health behaviours of adolescents. This may include interventions that target those close relationships which influence the sexual and reproductive experiences of adolescents, such as parents, intimate and other sexual partners, and peers.
- At the community level, there is a need to create positive social norms and community support for adolescents to practise safer behaviours and access SRH information and services. This involves interventions aimed at broader community members and institutions outside the family in neighbourhoods, schools and workplaces.
- At the societal level, there is a need to promote laws and policies related to the health, social, economic and educational spheres and to build broad societal norms in support of SRH and helping adolescents realize their human rights.[53]

In practical terms, these arenas require myriad initiatives—related to or in coordination with formal SRH infrastructures—all with the purpose of lowering young people's sexual and reproductive risk profiles, either directly (counselling; life skills and vocational training; other forms of economic empowerment for girls; partner-oriented programmes) and indirectly (incentives to remain in school; peer support groups; engaging men and boys in gender awareness training; involvement of adults and community leaders). As one review of the literature concluded, 'The sexual and reproductive health needs of adolescents are severely underserved and the provision of youth-friendly services alone is not sufficient to meet them. Supply side interventions needs to be combined with demand side activities to create a more supportive environment for adolescent care seeking and increased uptake of services, and governments need to work in partnership with civil society and community organizations to reach young people effectively.'[54]

However, no single initiative is likely to be revelatory, wholly successful or very widely applicable without adjustment to local circumstances. The subjective aspects of human sexuality are remarkably varied and the formative influences on adolescent identity and behaviours can be identified in broad terms but are expressed in countless ways throughout sub-Saharan Africa. The pressures to design, implement, monitor and evaluate programmes to improve adolescent sexual and reproductive health are urgent and considerable, as one broad survey study indicated: 'Many of the limitations encountered [in increasing SRH demand and community support] point to the pressing need for further research on how to best deliver adolescent SRH intervention packages and determine which components are most effective. Cost-effectiveness analyses and even cost data were largely unavailable. Fiscal responsibility and constrained budgets demand research to determine the best buys to improve adolescent SRH.'[55]

Issues

Contraception and Abortion

Practically everywhere, contraception and abortion share points of convergence between self-determining individual choice, intimate relations, law, religion, morality and politics. They are critical inflection points in sexual and reproductive health and they exist in complex relational patterns with one another, not only at the individual level but also in terms of the wider currents of global health, national health policies and donor funding, all of which have a formative effect on both subjective experience and medical objectivity.

The difficulty of obtaining reliable statistical indicators for behaviours that can variously be illegal (in the case of abortion), undertaken by 'hiding' populations (such as sex workers), that contravene local norms (unmarried adolescents) or breach the felt boundaries of privacy means that although there are observable demographic trends and statistics from abortion clinics where these are legal, it is difficult to get a full and detailed snapshot of the extent of abortion—and still more of the forms of reasoning which shape decision-making. We are better placed on the extent of contraceptive use and the methods adopted.[56] 'Data on the use of contraception have become increasingly available, but in many countries they are still only available for women of reproductive age (15–49 years) who are married or in a union. [However], countries in sub-Saharan Africa have the best coverage of survey data on contraceptive methods with more than two thirds of survey-based observations coming from either Demographic and Health Surveys (DHS) or Multiple Indicator Cluster Surveys (MICS).'[57] Another notable finding is that although religious strictures also have a role in setting the contraceptive 'climate,' the evidence suggests that religious affiliation is not a good predictor of behaviour in reproductive matters, since conformity with declared doctrine is often subject to local and personal circumstances.[58]

Contraception
Demographic trends and abortion statistics readily suggest that in much of SSA, the central difficulty for women trying to control their fertility is unmet need. Yet in addition to inequitable norms placing some women in a quandary between their wishes, those of their partners and prevailing expectations,[59] the term 'unmet need' filters out the subjective experiences of women who do not wish to become pregnant but who choose not to adopt modern contraceptive methods. The following summary of a 2016 Guttmacher Institute report explains:

> Most of the women [who wish to avoid pregnancy but do not use modern contraceptive methods] do not lack access to contraception but, rather, choose not to use it. Fewer than one in ten women categorised as having unmet need report that they are not aware of or cannot access a method of contraception. In countries across the developing world, the most common reasons for not using a method of contraception are perceived low risk of pregnancy (often due to infrequent sex or post-partum and lactational infecundity), a personal opposition to using contraception, and concerns about the health effects or side-effects of contraceptive use. For many women, the possibility of pregnancy seems remote, whereas the physical experience of using a contraceptive is immediate, tangible, and objectionable. For women who view themselves as being at low risk of pregnancy, use of early medical abortion for a rare unwanted pregnancy might be preferable to daily contraceptive use. Addressing the needs of the significant fraction of women (23 per cent of those with unmet need) who report personal or family opposition to using contraception and of those who feel that the side-effects of use outweigh the benefits (26 per cent of those with unmet need) requires thoughtful consideration of their concerns. A one-size-fits-all technological solution and a culture of family planning service delivery whose main aim is

to maximise the number of users, is unlikely to adequately address the personal, sexual, physical, and cultural aspects of contraceptive use. That health concerns and dislike of contraceptive side-effects are so common across countries indicates a need for development of new methods of contraception and a woman-centered approach to contraceptive provision.[60]

Another study confirms that what often passes for 'unmet need' is not a general unavailability of modern contraceptives but the absence of them in an acceptable form:

No single method serves the needs of every subgroup in a population. The one-method programs established by some ministries of health exclude many people interested in using family planning and tend to result in low proportions of the population using contraception. In such cases, the addition of another modern method to a program's method mix can raise total use. Adding more methods helps up to a point, until diminishing returns set in. All this depends partly upon which methods are offered, but the very presence of more choices can assist users whose needs could not be met by any single method.[61]

But the importance of contraception extends far beyond family planning because HIV looms over nearly every important element of sexual and reproductive health in sub-Saharan Africa, linking individual deliberation, health service priority-setting and patterns of donor funding. For example, 'The progress of family planning [...] began to stall in the early 1990s, perhaps due to the emerging threat of HIV/AIDS at that time, shifting global funding priorities: between 1992 and 2005, the percentage share of donor funding in the area of population sectors decreased from 32·1 per cent to 8 per cent. The donor financing for family planning was US$ 722·8 million in 1998 and was reduced to $393·5 million in 2006.'[62]

A notable trend in modern contraceptive use is the preponderance of injectable forms, typically several times greater than the use of male condoms in many sub-Saharan states, including several with relatively high HIV prevalence. According to the latest UN statistics, the percentage use of injectables to condoms is 4.3/1.1 (Nigeria); 17.6/2.3 (Uganda); 19.3/4.0 (Zambia); 23.9/8.8 (South Africa); and 30.0/1.9 in Malawi.[63] This is in a region with both the highest rates of new HIV infections as well as the highest rates of unintended pregnancies, although potential implications of hormonal contraceptives (including injectables) for transmission and progression of HIV is as yet unclear.[64]

The implications of HIV for contraception include the avoidance of transmission both directly through sexual relations between discordant individuals and mother-to-child infection—critically, because of a very large cohort of HIV-positive adolescents. 'With increased access to anti-retroviral treatment in sub-Saharan Africa, the number of children vertically infected with HIV who survive to adolescence has risen. Coupled with sustained high HIV-incidence among youth in the region, this has resulted in nearly 1.7 million HIV-positive adolescents (10–19 years old) in sub-Saharan Africa, with girls representing nearly two-thirds of this total. Despite global reductions in HIV prevalence, rates of new HIV infections remain the highest among 15–24 year old youth in sub-Saharan Africa. As their numbers continue to grow, adolescents and youth living with HIV are an essential group for secondary HIV prevention efforts.'[65]

HIV is not the only point at which the role of contraception in sexual health intersects with reproductive health, most dramatically in the intermittent (and current) reinstatement of the US Global Gag Rule, under which foreign NGOs cannot receive funding from the US government for family planning services if they also provide education, information, advice or counselling on abortion. The most recent imposition of what is sometimes referred to as the 'Mexico City policy' first initiated in 1984 is much wider in scope, with alarming implications that include but extend beyond core reproductive health services in many of the world's poorest states. 'Under [President] Trump's order, the gag rule now applies not only to US bilateral family planning assistance (US$575 million for fiscal year 2016), but also to all "global health assistance furnished by all departments or agencies"—encompassing an estimated $9.5 billion in foreign aid. Foreign NGOs that receive US funding to work on a broad range of health programmes in about 60 low-income and middle-income countries—including on HIV/AIDS, the Zika virus, malaria, tuberculosis, nutrition, and maternal and child health, among others—will potentially be subject to the same ideological restrictions that have hampered family planning aid at points in the past. Thus, President Trump's version of the global gag rule represents a wider attack on global health aid writ large.'[66] The grim irony in this and previous impositions of the gag rule is that it might have led to an increase in the number of abortions.[67]

Abortion

As an issue, abortion cannot be entirely abstracted from the availability, affordability and acceptability of reliable contraceptive methods. Nor can it be reduced to a small number of binaries—aborting/carrying a foetus to term; legal/illegal; safe/unsafe. Instead, it is at the centre of a tangled network of conditions and sub-issues before and after the fact which shape deliberation and risk calculation, together with consequences and costs ranging from the deeply personal to the social and political. Major themes identified in a survey of the literature include: adolescent sexual and reproductive health (unmet needs, delay of marriage); decentralization of abortion services to primary level (feasibility, innovations); legal restrictions and reforms and their impact on unsafe abortion and maternal mortality; unwanted pregnancies and the (non-) use of contraceptives; inequity in access to abortion services (rural/urban, rich/poor); male and female perspectives on abortion and gender imbalances in reproductive health decision-making (beliefs; link with gender-based violence); differences between first and second trimester abortions; the costs of unsafe abortion (individual, household, health system, societal); post-abortion care (counselling and contraceptive methods); methods and reasons for women self-inducing abortions; health worker and community attitudes towards abortions; and changing lifestyles and demand for abortion services. It appears that the degree to which abortion is legally sanctioned/restricted throughout sub-Saharan Africa is a key determinant for the fact that the number of abortions in that region (and, indeed, throughout the developing world) has changed remarkably little since 1990. According to the Guttmacher Institute, 'As of 2010–2014, an estimated 36 abortions occur each year per 1,000 women aged 15–44 in developing regions, compared with 27 in developed regions. The abortion rate declined significantly in developed regions since 1990–1994; however, no significant change occurred in developing regions.' Notably, the report indicates that 'abortions occur as frequently in the two most-restrictive categories of countries (banned outright or allowed only to save the woman's life) as in the least-restrictive category (allowed without restriction as to reason)—37 and 34 per 1,000 women, respectively.'[68]

The following list recognizes six categories of restricted abortion allowance in the countries of sub-Saharan Africa, with the third and following categories making at least some further allowances for cases of rape, incest and foetal abnormality (Table 4.1).

Yet even in South Africa where abortion has been legal since 1996, unsafe abortions persist for a variety of reasons—not least that on one estimate 30 per cent of South African women do not know that they have a right to legal, safe abortions.[69] Other factors include the risk of social

Table 4.1 Restrictions on abortion in the countries of sub-Saharan Africa

1. **Prohibited altogether (no explicit legal exceptions):** Angola, Congo-Brazzaville Congo-Kinshasa, Gabon, Guinea-Bissau, Madagascar Mauritania, Sao Tome and Principe, Senegal.
2. **To save the life of a woman:** Côte d'Ivoire, Libya, Malawi, Mali, Nigeria, Somalia, South Sudan, Tanzania, Uganda
3. **To save life of a woman/preserve physical health:** Ethiopia, Guinea, Kenya Lesotho, Niger, Rwanda, Togo, Zimbabwe
4. **To save life of a woman/ preserve physical/mental health:** Botswana, Eritrea, Gambia, Ghana, Liberia, Mozambique, Namibia Sierra Leone, Swaziland
5. **To save life of a woman/preserve physical/mental health/on socio-economic grounds:** Zambia
6. **No restriction as to reason (with gestational and other requirements):** South Africa

Adapted from Susheella Singh et al., 'Abortion Worldwide 2017: Uneven Progress and Unequal Access,' report from the Guttmacher Institute (March 2018), available at: https://www.guttmacher.org/report/abortion-worldwide-2017]

stigma when abortion clinics are stand-alone rather than integrated into larger family planning or general health clinics; declared conscientious objection by some health staff; lack of access; and in what bears similarities with the loss of momentum behind HIV prevention once antiretrovirals became widely available,

> The collapse of all but one of the women's health advocacy groups that had built national support for the development, passing, and implementation of the [1996 legalization of abortion] is indicative of the overarching reproductive health landscape. [...] Activism and advocacy lost momentum after the passage of the law, [although] it is necessary to keep the conversation on safe abortion, and maintain pressure on the Department of Health [DOH] to keep implementation moving. This lack of political will in the DOH manifested in an overreliance on international NGOs for some regions and services, a state of affairs interviewees felt to be unsustainable: "there have to be national competencies to ensure provincial and local implementation."[70]

Responding to the Difficult SRH Contexts in Sub-Saharan Africa

The fundamentals of sexual and reproductive health in sub-Saharan Africa differ little from those that pertain elsewhere in the world: the ability of girls and women to control their fertility, have sufficient knowledge to be able to do so; have affordable access to the necessary services; and to be able to have the means to be self-determining within the sexual relationships they contract. Much of this cannot be fully enabled without the corollary—male sexual health and gender attitudes—since a considerable amount of the preventable harm in the sexual and reproductive realms turns on the quality of relations in which the male prerogative is so often predominant. There is, in addition, the lesbian, gay, bisexual and transgender (LGBTQ) community, whose needs and vulnerabilities typically manifest in repressive circumstances. Their struggles restore not only the larger heterosexual community but also the framers of public policy to the importance of health rights. The brief consideration of contraception and abortion (above) makes clear that in the movement from rights/citizen entitlements to SRH provision, there is often a considerable distance between objective, medical assessments of needs, and the subjective experiences, perceptions and preferences of individuals. LGBTQ individuals seeking information, counselling or SRH services will feel this acutely, so research conducted on their values, attitudes and behaviours is much to be welcomed,[71] as is the performance of health systems and medical staffs in addressing their needs.[72]

On the basis of this chapter's survey of SRH contexts and issues, we can view the prospect with some degree of optimism, but we should not confuse ringing governmental endorsements for actionable agendas and be sceptical about quick transformations of social norms or addressing myriad human particulars with strategically driven and enacted initiatives; and recognize that there is no escape from politics—which includes the vagaries of public and private foreign donor funding.

The Map Is Not the Territory

The abundance of data, the extent of at least feasibly preventable suffering and the urgency of many of the worst conditions with their attendant vulnerabilities has galvanized sub-Saharan African states and the international community—certainly at the level of formal, outline commitments. The point here is not merely that an aspiration is not an agenda but that even the best planned SRH initiatives can falter for many reasons: because the funding is not sustainable; because the on-the-ground reality is often replete with unforeseen human particulars and complications; because existing health infrastructures are not sufficiently extensive, embedded and coherent to deliver their remits to a high standard, consistently; because political willingness is never sufficient on its own; because local forms of connectedness, knowledge and advocacy are not engaged or sometimes lost to high-profile programmes; because human systems are inherently inefficient; because particular issues are not always a simple matter to abstract from their contexts in order to address them directly—a list that could easily be extended from almost any point in the broad sexual and reproductive health rights (SRHR) literature.

At the same time, substantial progress has been made in many of the key indicators of sexual and reproductive health. For example, between 2007 and 2016, the African under-five mortality rate decreased from 98.1 to 69.7 per 1000 live births; and the infant mortality rate in Africa dropped significantly in the same period, from 63.5 to 46.3 deaths per 1000 newborns. Largely (though not throughout the whole of SSA), fertility rates have declined, and contraceptive options have become more readily available.

Social norms can and do alter, but they cannot be engineered; and subjectivities, although difficult to predict and pinpoint, can offer useful insights into tailoring or at least widening services and interventions appropriately

Social norms vary in their extent, inclusiveness and strength; and culture, tradition, peer pressure, sanctions for non-conformity all play a part in maintaining them against challenges and changing conditions. The larger social norms with a bearing on SRH often have a strong moral element, whether expressed in explicit terms or as long-standing traditions/taboos; and they are largely impervious to human rights claims. For this reason, health human rights advocacy needs to be deployed deftly, with a sensitivity to the political challenges involved in having human rights as an idea and ideal expressed as public policy through a government's political machinery—and with some thought given to the aftermath, since the passage of innovative SRH law is a threshold, not the arena. (The collapse of public advocacy after South Africa's legalization of abortion with consequent impacts on uptake, accessibility and quality of service provision (cited above) is a case in point.)

Adolescent sexuality is particularly difficult to comprehend and track in a systematic way, but it is not unique in respect of subjective perceptions and felt needs that can fall outside of the services and programmes designed to deal with problems most readily grasped in aggregate terms. While work to continue refining interventions remains important, the concept of Holistic Sexuality Education (HSE) is being developed. 'It is not an intervention, but a learning process, that starts from a holistic concept of (sexual) well-being, and goes beyond public health. It is a long-term process, involving many stake-holders, starting early in life and is spread out in an age- and developmentally appropriate way throughout childhood and adolescence. It does not try to change sexual behavior, rather it wants to enable people to, ultimately, achieve a safe and satisfactory sexual life.'[73] This can surely be regarded as a form of normative change, likely to be enduring.

Open Access

Broader trends in development throughout SSA can also drive normative change with positive SRH outcomes—and these were certainly a driver for the positive health outcomes of the Millennium Development Goals, furthering and facilitating the SDG targets. These trends have not ceased. For example, 'Social structures in sub-Saharan African countries are changing, and, despite the observed heterogeneity, there is growing evidence of the impact of the structural changes that customarily accompany socioeconomic development, urbanization, and normative change through mass media exposure and geographic mobility. In particular, the establishment of linked mobile telecommunication networks throughout the region and the rapid increase in cell and smart phone access are accelerating the spread of information and ideas, especially among young people. This includes information on sexual and reproductive health, methods of contraception, and abortion. Social change is also eroding traditional practices of postpartum abstinence, common in Western Africa.'[74] (In 2016, Botswana, Gabon, South Africa, Gambia and Ghana all had more mobile subscriptions per inhabitant than the EU average.)

Urgent needs *set against constrained funding mean that hard choices cannot be avoided*

The largest, limiting contexts for progressing sexual and reproductive health in sub-Saharan African states are neither epidemiological nor programmatic, but are grounded in the priorities of donor states and the competing health demands of all states, both within and beyond SSA. This is clear in the costings for Sustainable Development Goal 3, 'Ensure healthy lives and promote wellbeing for all at all ages,' which are not realistically achievable. To begin, the wider SDG context is instructive. It has been estimated that the additional costs for the entire SDG agenda in lower- and middle-income countries would be at least $1.4 trillion per year—six times net official development assistance for the entire world. Even setting aside a range of political pressures and calculations, it is not plausible to suppose that those sums will readily be forthcoming, on any combination of recipient countries assuming a higher share of the burdens and/or donor countries disbursing considerably greater funds. So hard choices await—or some goals and targets will fail by default—and there is no reason to assume that some health targets will not be amongst them.

We can hope that economic and social improvements in some countries will register on key SDG health indicators by dint of improving the social determinants of health, but not under the direct aegis of the SDGs. Yet with sufficient impetus from state and regional leaderships and from donors, it will be possible to reduce the global maternal mortality ratio to less than 70 per 100,000 live births—an important SDG health goal. And there are other health targets that are similarly within the bounds of the possible.

However, SDG 3 also determines 'by 2030, [to] end the epidemics of AIDS, tuberculosis, malaria and neglected tropical diseases and combat hepatitis, water-borne diseases and other communicable diseases.' But note that Millennium Development Goal Target 6.A was 'to have halted and begun to reverse the spread of HIV/AIDS,' and Target 6.B was to have achieved, 'by 2010, universal access to treatment for HIV/AIDS for all those who need it.' We managed neither: the rate of new HIV infections remains alarmingly high (at something like 1.8 million), and of the estimated 36 million people infected, only 55 per cent are receiving antiretrovirals.

Of the wider SDG3, WHO has estimated that it will require between an additional $274 billion (the 'progress' scenario) and $371 billion (the 'ambitious' scenario) per year. A $20–54 billion per year funding gap is projected. Even if we accept that these cost estimates are accurate and achievable, what then? The penultimate SDG target commits us in the broadest terms to 'substantially increase health financing and the recruitment, development, training and retention of the health workforce in developing countries, especially in least developed countries and small island developing States.' What might this amount to? A 2017 WHO study[75] specifies that its 'ambitious' scenario would add more than 23.6 million health workers, 3 million of whom would be medical doctors, and includes the construction of 415, 000 health facilities, of which 378,000 would be primary health centres. But quantifying human and material resources to match identified needs does not transform an aspiration into a strategy. No amount of funding will train 3 million doctors over the next 10 years: the conditions will not support the ambition. Hard choices await—not only for the SDGs as a whole, but in all likelihood, also for its ambitious health targets.

What the countries of sub-Saharan Africa can achieve—alone, through regional organization and with the help of the international community is addressed in the next chapter.

NOTES

1. Markus Haacker, *The Economics of the Global Response to HIV/AIDS* (Oxford: Oxford University Press, 2016), Chapter 5.
2. Ana Langer et al., 'Women and health: the key for sustainable development,' (Lancet Commission), *Lancet* 386 (2015), pp. 1165–210, available at: https://doi.org/10.1016/S0140-6736(15)60497-4
3. African Union, *Agenda 2063: The Africa We Want* (April 2015), available at: https://www.un.org/en/africa/osaa/pdf/au/agenda2063.pdf
4. https://www.unfpa.org/sites/default/files/pub-pdf/programme_of_action_Web%20ENGLISH.pdf
5. For a brief chronology with citations to primary documents, see UN Women, 'World Conferences on Women,' available at: https://www.unwomen.org/en/how-we-work/intergovernmental-support/world-conferences-on-women
6. ICPD Beyond 2014 International Conference on Human Rights, Conference Report, (2013), pp. 31–2, available at: https://www.ohchr.org/Documents/Issues/Women/WRGS/ICP_%20Beyond_2014_International_Thematic_Conference/Report_of_the_ICPD_Beyond_2014_International_Conference_on_Human_Rights.pdf
7. African Union Commission, 'Sexual and Reproductive Health and Rights: Continental Policy Framework' (2005), available at: https://au.int/sites/default/files/documents/30921-doc-srhr_english_0.pdf
8. African Union Commission, Maputo Plan of Action 2016–30 and Reproductive Health Services In Africa for The Operationalisation of the Continental Policy Framework for Sexual and Reproductive Health and Rights, available at: https://au.int/sites/default/files/newsevents/workingdocuments/27514-wd-mpoa_7-_revised_au_stc_inputs_may_se-rob-director_002.pdf
9. Bob Mwiinga Munyati, 'African women's sexual and reproductive health and rights: The revised Maputo Plan of Action pushes for upscaled delivery,' *Agenda: Empowering Women for Gender Equity* Vol. 32(1) (2018), pp. 36–45

10. John Cleland, 'Contraception and health,' *The Lancet* Vol. 380 (14 July 2012), pp. 149–52.

11. Olena Ivanova, Masna Rai and Elizabeth Kemigisha, 'A Systematic Review of Sexual and Reproductive Health Knowledge, Experiences and Access to Services among Refugee, Migrant and Displaced Girls and Young Women in Africa,' *International Journal of Environmental Research and Public Health 15*, (2018), doi: https://doi.org/10.3390/ijerph15081583

12. Blessing Mberu, et al., 'Bringing Sexual and Reproductive Health in the Urban Contexts to the Forefront of the Development Agenda: The Casefor Prioritizing the Urban Poor,' *Maternal and* Child *Health Journal* 18(2), (September 2014), pp. 1572–77.

13. Miriam Hartmann, et al., 'How Are Gender Equality and Human Rights Interventions Included in Sexual and Reproductive Health Programmes and Policies: A Systematic Review of Existing Research Foci and Gaps,' PLoS ONE 11(12) (2016), DOI: https://doi.org/10.1371/jopurnal. pone.0167542

14. Ashley M. Fox, 'The Social Determinants of HIV Serostatus in Sub-Saharan Africa: An Inverse Relationship Between Poverty and HIV?' *Public Health Reports*, Supplement 4, Volume 125 (2010), p. 23. See also: M. Hajizadeh, et al. 'Socioeconomic inequalities in HIV/AIDS prevalence in sub-Saharan African countries: evidence from the Demographic Health Surveys,' *International Journal for Equity in Health* 13(18) (2014), doi: https://doi.org/10.1186/1475-9276-13-18

15. Anne Margreth Bakilana, '7 facts about population in Sub-Saharan Africa,' 29 October 2015, available at: http://blogs.worldbank.org/africacan/7-facts-about-population-in-sub-saharan-africa

16. Maria Dörnemann and Teresa Huhle, 'Population problems in modernization and development,' in The Population Knowledge Network (eds), *Twentieth Century Population Thinking: A Critical Reader of Primary Sources* (Abingdon: Routledge, 2015), pp. 142–72.

17. OECD, *Development Co-operation Report 2012: Lessons in Linking Sustainability* and Development, p. 71. Available at: https://www-oecd-ilibrary-org.ezp; see also: Michael Herrmann, 'Sustainable development, demography and sexual and reproductive health: inseparable linkages and their policy implications,' *Reproductive Health Matters*, Vol. 22, No. 43, (May 2014), pp. 28–42.

18. David Canning, Sangeeta Raja, and Abdo S. Yazbeck, eds, *Africa's Demographic Transition Dividend or Disaster?* World Bank (2015), available at: https://openknowledge.worldbank.org/handle/10986/22036

19. David Antonio Sanchez-Paez and Jose Antonio Ortega, 'Adolescent contraceptive use and its effects on fertility,' *Demographic Research*. Volume 38, Article 45 (2018), p. 1359. DOI: https://doi.org/10.4054/DemRes.2018.38.45

20. World Health Organization, Trends in maternal mortality 1990–2015, available at: https://www.who.int/reproductivehealth/publications/monitoring/maternal-mortality-2015/en/

21. The Lancet Infectious Diseases Commission (9 July 2017), p. e235.

22. Rachel Sullivan Robinson, Intimate interventions in global health : family planning and HIV prevention in sub-Saharan Africa (Cambridge: Cambridge University Press, 2017), p. 99.

23. Rachel Sullivan Robinson, *Intimate interventions in global health: family planning and HIV prevention in sub-Saharan Africa* (Cambridge: Cambridge University Press, 2017), p. 101.

24. Arin Dutta et al., 'The HIV Treatment Gap: Estimates of the Financial Resources Needed versus Available for Scale-Up of Antiretroviral Therapy in97 Countries from 2015 to 2020,' *PLoS Medicine* 12(11) (2015), doi:10.1371/ journal.pmed.1001907

25. Maureen Lewis and Marijn Verhoeven, 'Financial Crises and Social Spending: The Impact of the 2008–2009 Crisis,' World Bank (June 18, 2010), p. 12. Available at: https://openknowledge.worldbank.org/bitstream/handle/10986/12965/698780ESW0P0970370021B00PUBLIC00ACS.pdf?sequence=1&isAllowed=

26. Nana K. Poku, 'HIV Prevention: The key to ending AIDS by 2030,' *The Open AIDS Journal* 10 (2016), abstract, p. 65.

27. UNAIDS, 'Fact Sheet—Global AIDS Update, 2019,' available at: https://www.unaids.org/sites/default/files/media_asset/UNAIDS_FactSheet_en.pdf

28. The Law Library of Congress, Global Legal Research Center, 'Laws on Homosexuality in African Nations,' February 2014. Available at: https://www.loc.gov/law/help/criminal-laws-on-homosexuality/homosexuality-laws-in-african-nations.pdf

29. Amaya Perez-Brumer, Richard Parker and Peter Aggleton (eds), *Rethinking MSM, trans* and other categories in HIV prevention* (London: Routledge, 2018).

30. Alexandra Müller et al., '"You have to make a judgment call": Morals, judgments and the provision of quality sexual and reproductive health services for adolescents in South Africa,' *Social Science and Medicine* 148 (2016), pp. 71–8; Pamela M Godia, 'Sexual reproductive health service provision to young people in Kenya: health service providers' experiences,' *BMC Health Services Research* 13 (2013), available at: http://www.biomedcentral.com/1472-6963/13/476

31. D. M. Reddy, R. Fleming and C. Swain, 'Effect of mandatory parental notification on adolescent girls' use of sexual health care services,' *Journal of the American Medical Association* 288(6) (2002), pp. 710–14.

32. WHO, Adolescent HIV testing, counselling and care: Implementation guidance for health providers and planners: Key populations, available at: http://apps.who.int/adolescent/hiv-testing-treatment/page/key_ populations

33. R. M. Viner et al., 'Adolescence and the social determinants of health,' *Lancet* 379 (9826), (2012), pp. 1641–52.

34. World Health Organization, Multi-country study on women's health and domestic violence against women (2005), available at: https://www.who.int/reproductivehealth/publications/violence/24159358X/en/

35. King K. Holmeset et al. (eds), *Sexually Transmitted Diseases* (New York: McGraw-Hill, 2008), p. 155. See also: M. Laga et al. 'To stem HIV in Africa, prevent transmission to young women,' *AIDS*, 15(7) (2001), pp. 931–34.

36. For example, cash transfers for the purpose of vulnerability and risk reduction. See: L. Cluver et al., 'Child-focused state cash transfer and adolescent risk of HIV infection in South Africa: a propensity-score-matched case-control study,' *Lancet Global Health* 1(6) (2013), pp. e362–e370; A. Pettifor et al., 'Can money prevent the spread of HIV? A review of cash payments for HIV prevention,' *AIDS and Behavior* 16(7) (2012), pp. 1729–1738; S. Handa et al., 'The government of Kenya's cash transfer program reduces the risk of sexual debut among young people age 15–25,' *PLoS One* 9(1) (2014), doi: https://doi.org/10.1371/journal.pone.0085473; D. de Walque et al., 'Incentivising safe sex: a randomised trial of conditional cash transfers for HIV and sexually transmitted infection prevention in rural Tanzania,' *BMJ Open* 2 (2012), doi: https://doi.org/10.1136/bmjopen-2011-000747

37. Alissa Koski, Shelley Clark and Arijit Nandi, 'Has Child Marriage Declined in sub-Saharan Africa? An Analysis of Trends in 31 Countries,' *Population and Development Review* 43(1) (March 2017), p. 26.

38. Institute for Health Metrics, University of Washington, 'Financing Global Health 2017: Funding Universal Health Coverage and the Unfinished HIV/AIDS Agenda,' p. 77. Available at: http://www.healthdata.org/sites/default/files/files/policy_report/FGH/2018/IHME_FGH_2017_fullreport_online.pdf

39. Ibid.

40. Commission on Macroeconomics and Health, 'Macroeconomics and Health: Investing in Health for Economic Development,' WHO, 2001, available at: http://apps.who.int/iris/bitstream/10665/42435/1/924154550X.pdf; World Health Organization, Regional Office for Africa, 'Universal Health Coverage,' available at: https://www.afro.who.int/health-topics/universal-health-coverage

41. John Palen et al., 'PEPFAR, Health System Strengthening, and Promoting Sustainability and Country Ownership,' *Journal of Acquired Immune Deficiency Syndrome* 60 (2012), S113–S119.
42. Till Bärnighausen et al., 'Going Horizontal—Shifts in Funding of Global Health Intervention,' *The New England Journal of Medicine* 364 (2011), pp. 2181–83.
43. See for example: Global Fund, 35th Board Meeting, 'The Global Fund sustainability, transition and co-financing policy' (April 2016), available at: https://www.theglobalfund.org/media/4221/bm35_04-sustainabilitytransitionandcofinancing_policy_en.pdf.
44. George Gotsadze, 'The Challenges of Transition From Donor-Funded Programs: Results From a Theory-Driven Multi-Country Comparative Case Study of Programs in Eastern Europe and Central Asia Supported by the Global Fund,' *Global Health: Science and Practice*, Vol. 7(2) (2019), pp. 258–72.
45. Dvora Joseph Davey et al., 'Integrating Human Immunodeficiency Virus and Reproductive, Maternal and Child, and Tuberculosis Health ServicesWithin National Health Systems,' *Current HIV/AIDS Reports* 13(3), 170–76.
46. Mustapha D. Ibrahim et al., 'An Estimation of the Efficiency and Productivity of Healthcare Systems in Sub-Saharan Africa: Health-Centred Millennium Development Goal-Based Evidence,' *Social Indicators Research* 143(1) (May 2019), pp. 371–89.
47. UNFPA, Programme of Action adopted at the International Conference on Population and Development, 5–13 September 1994. Available at: https://unfpa.org/sites/default/files/event-pdf/PoA_en.pdf
48. WHO, 'Glion consultation on strengthening the linkages between reproductive health and HIV/AIDS,' WHO/HIV/2006.02 (2006). Available at: https://www.who.int/hiv/pub/advocacymaterials/glionconsultationsummary_DF.pdf; see also: WHO/UNFPOA/UNAIDS/IPPF, 'Sexual and Reproductive Health & HIV/AIDS: A Framework for Priority Linkages,' 2005. Available at: https://apps.who.int/iris/bitstream/handle/10665/69851/WHO_HIV_2005.05_eng.pdf;sequence=1
49. J. A. Smit et al., 'Key informant perspectives on policy and service level challenges and opportunities for delivering integrated sexual and reproductive health and HIV care in South Africa,' *BMC Health Services Research* 12   (2012),   doi: http://dx.doi.org.ezp.lib.cam.ac.uk/10.1186/1472-6963-12-48, pp. 7–8.
50. Claudia Garcia-Moreno et al., 'Prevalence of intimate partner violence: findings from the WHO multi-country study on women's health and domestic violence,' *The Lancet* 368(9543), (2006), pp. 1260–69.

51. UNAIDS, 'Women and HIV: A Spotlight on Adolescent Girls and Young Women' (2019), available at: https://www.unaids.org/sites/default/files/media_asset/2019_women-and-hiv_en.pdf

52. Venkatraman Chandra-Mouli et al., 'Twenty Years After the International Conference on Population and Development: Where Are We With Adolescent Sexual and Reproductive Health and Rights?' *Journal of Adolescent Health* 56 (2015), pp. S1–6.

53. Joar Svanemyr et al., 'Creating an Enabling Environment for Adolescent Sexual and Reproductive Health: A Framework and Promising Approaches,' *Journal of Adolescent Health* 56 (2015), p. S9.

54. Amy J. Kesterton and Meena Cabral de Mello, 'Generating demand and community support for sexual and reproductive health services for young people: A review of the Literature and Programs,' *Reproductive Health* 7:25 (2010), p. 10. Available at: http://www.reproductive-health-journal.com/content/7/1/25

55. Donna M. Denno et al., 'Effective Strategies to Provide Adolescent Sexual and Reproductive Health Services and to Increase Demand and Community Support,' *Journal of Adolescent Health* 56 (2015), p. S40. See also: Michelle J. Hindin et al., 'Setting research priorities for adolescent sexual and reproductive health in low- and middle-income countries,' *Bulletin of the World Health Organization*, 91(1) (January 2013), DOI: https://doi.org/10.2471/BLT.12.107565; WHO, Quality Assessment Handbook: A Guide to Assessing Health Services for Adolescent Clients' (2009). Available at: https://apps.who.int/iris/bitstream/handle/10665/44240/9789241598859_eng.pdf

56. Amy O Tsui, Win Brown and Qingfeng Li, 'Contraceptive Practice in sub-Saharan Africa,' *Population and Development Review* 43 (Supplement 1) (May 2017), pp. 166–91.

57. United Nations, Department of Economic and Social Affairs, 'Contraceptive Use by Method, 2019: Data Booklet,' p. 14. Available at: https://www.un.org/en/development/desa/population/publications/pdf/family/ContraceptiveUseByMethodDataBooklet2019.pdf

58. Victor Agadjanian, Lubayna Fawcett and Scott T. Yabiku, 'History, Community Milieu, and Christian-Muslim Differentials in Contraceptive Use in Sub-Saharan Africa,' *Journal for the Scientific Study of Religion* 48(3) (2009), pp. 462–79.

59. Nathalie Bajos et al., 'Normative Tensions and Women's Contraceptive Attitudes and Practices in Four African Countries,' *Population* 68(1) (2013), pp. 15–36.

60. Diana Greene Foster, 'Unmet need for abortion and woman-centred contraceptive care,' *The Lancet*, Vol. 388, Issue 10,041 (16–22 July 2016), p. 216; Gilda Sedgh, Lori S. Ashford and Rubina Hussain, 'Unmet Need for Contraception in Developing Countries: Examining Women's Reasons

for Not Using a Method,' The Guttmacher Institute (June 2016), available at: https://www.guttmacher.org/report/unmet-need-for-contraception-in-developing-countries

61. John Ross and John Stover, 'Use of modern contraception increases when more methods become available: analysis of evidence from 1982–2009,' *Global Health: Science and Practice* 1(2) (August 2013), p. 203.

62. Saifuddin Ahmed et al., 'Trends in contraceptive prevalence rates in sub-Saharan Africa since the 2012 London Summit on Family Planning: result from repeated cross-sectional surveys,' *Lancet Global Health* 7 (17 May 2019), p. e905.

63. United Nations, Department of Economic and Social Affairs, *World Contraceptive Use 2018*, available at: https://www.un.org/en/development/desa/population/publications/dataset/contraception/wcu2018.asp

64. C. B. Polis, et al., 'An updated systematic review of epidemiological evidence on hormonal contraceptive methods and HIV acquisition in women,' *AIDS* 30 (2016), pp. 2665–83; R. Heffron, et al., 'Use of hormonal contraceptives and risk of HIV-1 transmission: A prospective cohort study,' *Lancet Infectious Disease* 12(1) (2012), pp. 19–26.

65. Eloina Toska et al., 'Sex in the shadow of HIV: A systematic review of prevalence, risk factors, and interventions to reduce sexual risk-taking among HIV-positive adolescents and youth in sub-Saharan Africa,' *PLOS One* 12(6) (2017), p. 2.

66. *The Lancet* (Comment), 'The Trump global gag rule: an attack on US family planning and global health aid,' Vol. 389 (4 February 2017), p. 485.

67. Eran Bendavid et al., 'United States aid policy and induced abortion in sub-Saharan Africa,' *Bulletin of the World Health Organization*, Vol. 89(12) (01 December 2011), pp. 873-880C; Nina Brooks et al., 'USA aid policy and induced abortion in sub-Saharan Africa: an analysis of the Mexico City Policy,' *The Lancet Global Health* 7(8) (2019), pp. 1046e–1053.

68. Susheella Singh et al., 'Abortion Worldwide 2017: Uneven Progress and Unequal Access,' report from the Guttmacher Institute (March 2018), available at: https://www.guttmacher.org/report/abortion-worldwide-2017

69. Marie Stopes South Africa, 'Reproductive Health Rights in South Africa,' available at: https://www.mariestopes.org.za/reproductive-health-rights-in-south-africa/

70. Mary Favier et al., 'Safe abortion in South Africa: "We have wonderful laws but we don't have people to implement those laws",' *Gynecology and Obstetrics* 143(S4) (October 2018), pp. 42–3.

71. Valerie Rubinsky and Angela Cooke-Jackson, 'Sex as an Intergroup Arena: How Women and Gender Minorities Conceptualize Sex, Sexuality, and Sexual Health,' *Communication Studies* 69(2) (2018), pp. 213–34; Maxime Charest et al., 'Sexual health information disparities between heterosexual and LGBTQ+ young adults: Implications for sexual health,' *The Canadian Journal of Human Sexuality* 25(2) (2016), pp. 74–85.

72. R. E. Knight et al., 'Examining clinicians' experiences providing sexual health services for LGBTQ youth: considering social and structural determinants of health in clinical practice,' *Health Education Research* 29(4) (2014) pp. 662–70.

73. Kristien Michielsen et al., 'Reorienting adolescent sexual and reproductive health research: reflections from an international conference,' *Reproductive Health* 13(3) (2016), p. 2.

74. Amy O Tsui, Win Brown and Qingfeng Li, 'Contraceptive Practice in sub-Saharan Africa,' *Population and Development Review* 43 (Supplement 1) (May 2017), p. 187.

75. World Health Organization, 'WHO estimates cost of reaching global health targets by 2030,' 17 July 2017, available at: https://www.who.int/news-room/detail/17-07-2017-who-estimates-cost-of-reaching-global-health-targets-by-2030

CHAPTER 5

Challenges, Progress and Prospects

Abstract In many parts of sub-Saharan Africa, declaratory commitment to sexual and reproductive health rights faces very considerable policy-making conundrums which are reviewed in this chapter. These are most visible in the tensions emerging between the impetus for Universal Health Coverage and the ongoing struggle against HIV and AIDS. The opportunities being developed through African regional bodies are then considered, after which the challenges, progress and prospects for sexual and reproductive health rights in sub-Saharan Africa are reviewed in thematic form.

Keywords Universal Health Coverage • HIV • Rights • Norms

Policy-Making Conundrums

The largest and most important advances in sexual and reproductive health (SRH) in sub-Saharan Africa (SSA) can be made by preventive means. Specifically, social determinants largely create and sustain the conditions for SRH vulnerabilities, ill health and avoidable deaths. This is not to deny agency to those worst-placed to protect themselves and their loved ones, but to recognize that the relationships between poverty and SRH risk are

© The Author(s), under exclusive license to Springer Nature   93
Singapore Pte Ltd. 2020
N. K. Poku, *Sexual and Reproductive Health and Rights in
Sub-Saharan Africa*, Global Research in Gender, Sexuality and
Health, https://doi.org/10.1007/978-981-15-8502-9_5

not merely a matter of statistical correlation; that our failure to match the roll-out of antiretrovirals with concomitant HIV prevention means that AIDS is still an epidemic; and that because gender inequality is both endemic and embedded, its health consequences cannot be addressed by health systems alone, however well-funded and coherent they might be. The evidence is abundant—for example: 'In 51 countries with data on the subject, only 57 per cent of women aged 15 to 49, married or in union, make their own decisions about sexual relations and the use of contraceptives and health services.'[1]

At national and international levels, these and related points are not only acknowledged but proclaimed as commitments. For instance, Sustainable Development Goal (SDG) 5 ('Achieve gender equality and empower all women and girls') includes the following targets:

- End all forms of discrimination against all women and girls everywhere.
- Eliminate all forms of violence against all women and girls in the public and private spheres, including trafficking and sexual and other types of exploitation.
- Eliminate all harmful practices, such as child, early and forced marriage and female genital mutilation.

The list of commitments with a specific focus or direct bearing on SRH is contained in the following targets from Sustainable Development Goal 5 ('Ensure healthy lives and promote well-being for all at all ages'):

- By 2030, reduce the global maternal mortality ratio to less than 70 per 100,000 live births.
- By 2030, ensure universal access to sexual and reproductive health-care services, including for family planning, information and education, and the integration of reproductive health into national strategies and programmes.
- By 2030, end preventable deaths of newborns and children under 5 years of age, with all countries aiming to reduce neonatal mortality to at least as low as 12 per 1000 live births and under-5 mortality to at least as low as 25 per 1000 live births.
- By 2030, end the epidemics of AIDS, tuberculosis, malaria and neglected tropical diseases and combat hepatitis, water-borne diseases and other communicable diseases.

- Achieve universal health coverage, including financial risk protection, access to quality essential health-care services and access to safe, effective, quality and affordable essential medicines and vaccines for all.
- Substantially increase health financing and the recruitment, development, training and retention of the health workforce in developing countries, especially in least developed countries and small island developing States.
- Strengthen the capacity of all countries, in particular developing countries, for early warning, risk reduction and management of national and global health risks.

These targets are very considerable on any reckoning, not only for their breadth and the short timeline to 2030 for several of them, but also, as outlined in Chap. 4, because the vast scope of the SDGs makes it unlikely that any of the 'big ticket' goals and targets will enjoy consistent political support or sustained funding even on their own, much less in competitive standing with others. Currently, concerted action to halt climate change at both national and international levels is the most visible indicator of this.

At the same time, however, neither human health in general nor SRH in particular have a fixed place in a hierarchy of meaning or urgency. Governments in sub-Saharan Africa (as elsewhere) are sensitive to widely shared health concerns for both humane and self-interested reasons. These can range from issues of equity to the surge in non-communicable diseases. But few if any of these can be dealt with in a linear fashion, as though the largest part of what is required is that first, a preventable or treatable health condition accrues a critical mass of numbers and/or meaning to become a political matter—and from there, to policy-making, funding and implementation. The complex interconnectedness of human and environmental factors which shape and drive disease epidemiology are not a straight-forward fit with the policy-making machinery of states—demonstrated by persistent difficulties in determining the most effective prevention strategies for HIV and AIDS in SSA, despite the very considerable political and financial resources that have been devoted to it. In addition to the complexities, competition for political attention and finite resources are also operative. 'Policy formulation studies have demonstrated that social determinants are hard to act on in conventional policy-making environments because they are complex. This is especially difficult because the [social determinants of health] (SDH) agenda competes for policy attention with problems that are more straightforward and do not carry the demand for complex, multifaceted responses implicit in the evidence on SDH.'[2]

The broad social determinants of human health are not difficult to list—environmental quality, housing, nutrition and levels of employment feature as a matter of course, though notably, a dedicated consideration of gender, so central to SRH, is often missing.[3] But establishing causal relations between both environmental and human relational factors and health outcomes requires dedicated research to reveal in what ways, by what pathways, and to what degrees social constructs 'determine' specific health outcomes.[4] Similar difficulties attend our understanding of the ways in which poverty is also socially determined. A great deal of empirical research is still required to understand how both policy-making machinery and medical services can best be aligned to alleviate the egregious and closely linked conditions of poverty and ill health.[5]

Sub-Saharan Africa is beset by both, but although the aggregate statistics, both positive and negative, give a sense of the landscape, the challenges and prospects for the nations which comprise SSA and for the sub-groups within them vary quite considerably. Note, for example, that '[h]alf of Africa's poor live in 5 countries; and 10 countries [all of them sub-Saharan] account for 75 per cent of Africa's poor. Yet the poorest countries, and regions within countries (those with the highest poverty rates), are not necessarily the same countries or regions housing most of the poor. This poses a challenge as to where to target the poverty-reduction efforts, at least from a global perspective.'[6]

According to the latest World Bank analyses, 'Poverty in Africa has fallen substantially—from 54 per cent in 1990 to 41 per cent in 2015—but the number of poor has increased, from 278 million in 1990 to 413 million in 2015.' The declining percentage set against the substantial rise in absolute numbers of people living in poverty marks the key importance of sexual and reproductive health as essential to development. As the World Bank report concludes, 'With a total fertility rate of 4.8 births per woman, Africa is the fastest growing continent (2.7 per cent per year) and its demographic transition is slow. Rapid population growth and high fertility in many countries in Sub-Saharan Africa hold back poverty reduction in several ways. It will be critical for African countries to *accelerate the fertility transition,* through cost-effective interventions like family planning programs, which complement efforts to increase female education and increase their income opportunities for greater empowerment. With fewer children, families and governments will have the opportunity to invest more in each child's human capital.'[7]

Although the poverty trajectories for sub-Saharan Africa mean that it will not reach the SDG goal of eradicating poverty by 2030, more positive developments, fuelled by robust economic growth through the 1990s have ensured substantial, if very uneven progress across many of the most important development indicators, as the outcome of the Millennium Development Goals (MDGs) indicated. But accounting for the inconsistencies and the puzzle over which initiatives and which dynamics were 'determining' in one or more senses remains difficult to discern:

> The variation in outcomes during the MDG era prompts a question of why—what drove the differences? If one presumes, for example, that economic growth is the primary driver of outcomes, then one would need to substantiate how the same underlying patterns of growth led to such different trends across outcomes such as HIV/AIDS deaths, child mortality, primary school completion, and access to drinking water. Similarly, a hypothesis that commodity prices drove gains among low-income exporting economies would need to identify the pathways between commodity-specific price trends and the cross-section of relevant MDG indicator outcomes. Conversely, if one believes that official development assistance is a primary driver of specific results in low-income environments, then one would need to substantiate the links between issue-specific outcomes and relevant forms of public and private finance.[8]

From a regional perspective, the kinds, degrees and distribution of poverty throughout SSA render impractical any clear and broadly applicable characterization of it as a determinant of health—that requires more narrowly delineated, place- or population-specific studies that trace the relationships between poverty and epidemiology. What we can say is that there is a poverty-development-SRH nexus in sub-Saharan Africa which finds countless expressions in the tensions and hard choices which arise in the yawning gaps between needs and resources. That nexus is also the formative background to how the SSA region and its states conceptualize and prioritize SRH issues; how they balance any particular focus against other pressing matters and whether/how they can maximize positive outcomes from their investments and interventions, based on an appreciation of complex causal relations; and how they secure and maintain the necessary funding. The same broad set of considerations also concern both private and public donors; and although the purposes and priorities of external actors are not always entirely consonant with those of host states, scarce resources in the face of urgent necessity is compelling.

The Organization and Funding of Health Service Provision for SRH

Much as with health rights and gender equality, the importance of health systems that are well-funded and staffed, affordable, accessible and effective has received validation in national and international commitments as well as studies over many years. The good faith of the commitments can be taken at face value, but in practical terms, they are generally more aspirational than programmatic—and in the African Union's (AU's) *Africa 2063*, although gender equality is a specific goal, 'health' is only given 'nutrition' as its priority area; and there is no mention of health systems.[9] It might have been hoped that by 2063, AIDS will have receded sufficiently to be embedded within the normal range of health systems functioning—and indeed, that the region's health systems will be able to cater adequately for the burgeoning SRH needs of its youthful demographic as it lives through its sexual maturity.

But transitioning to largely AIDS-free populations in Sub-Saharan Africa and securing the necessary health service provision for their sexual and reproductive needs is a very large challenge—and each conditions the other because HIV and AIDS remain at the centre not only of sexual and reproductive health but also of SSA health systems and the question of how they can more effectively address the pandemic while simultaneously accommodating the demands for health systems of wider reach and inclusiveness.

HIV/AIDS and Universal Health Coverage

Although only five SSA states have an HIV prevalence rate in double digits, relatively low country-level figures mask alarmingly high rates in key populations, which means that the risk of a more generalized spread of the virus is always present. 'In Burundi, HIV prevalence in sex workers is 26.5 per cent compared to 1.0 per cent in the general adult population, whilst in Côte d'Ivoire amongst MSM and sex workers, HIV prevalence is 18.8 per cent and 28.7 per cent respectively compared to 2.7 per cent in the general adult population. To prevent epidemics expanding to the general population, HIV prevention efforts should focus on understanding the dynamics of HIV transmission, tracking the size and course of the epidemic and prioritizing and intensifying interventions in affected sub-populations.'[10]

In many ways, the HIV response over the past 30 years has been a trailblazer in global public health.[11] It has mobilized political figures, the international community, donors, health care providers, civil society, academia and the private sector around a common purpose. It has stimulated unprecedented investments in health and has played an important role in shaping the global health and development architecture. It has catalysed major breakthroughs in science and technology, including revitalizing infectious disease epidemiology and clinical management, creating a platform to tackle other newly emerging pathogens, such as Severe Acute Respiratory Syndrome (SARS) and the H5N1 Avian Influenza virus. It has demonstrated the feasibility of rapidly scaling up clinical and public health programmes in challenging environments and inspired new models of service delivery, such as decentralized and integrated services, task shifting and sharing, and inter-sectoral collaboration. It has additionally resulted in increased numbers of better trained health workers.[12] Moreover, it has demonstrated the importance of engaging communities and advocates in decision-making processes and highlighted their role in strengthening accountability mechanisms and championing affordable access to treatment and care.

However, the decline in recent years of the 'AIDS exceptionalism' argument that had marked the MDG era has manifested in the growing normative momentum behind the principle of Universal Health Coverage (UHC), which proposes to incorporate the HIV biomedical response into a package of essential health-care services, along with other contenders such as tuberculosis, malaria, non-communicable diseases, maternal and child health, which should be universally accessible and affordable. As the World Health Organization (WHO) defines it, 'Universal Health Coverage ensures that all people can use the promotive, preventive, curative, rehabilitative and palliative health services they need, of sufficient quality to be effective, while also ensuring that the use of these services does not expose the user to financial hardship.'[13]

The Global Drive Towards Universal Health Coverage

A dedicated network of 587 international non-governmental organizations, academic institutions and advocacy groups, supported by the Rockefeller Foundation, is behind the global push for Universal Health Coverage, which has culminated in Sustainable Development Goal 3.8: 'Achieve universal health coverage, including financial risk protection, access to quality essential health care services, and access to safe, effective, quality, and affordable essential medicines and vaccines for all.'[14] Importantly for the HIV response, UHC is predicated on the existence or development of 'a strong, efficient, well-run health system that meets priority health needs through people-centred integrated care.'[15] As such, the UHC approach would see the transition of the HIV response from a vertical programming approach, to being fully integrated with national health systems. The rationales for this are numerous, from leveraging HIV financing and the wealth of expertise, systems and processes it has accrued in order to strengthen broader health systems and services to address other essential health concerns; to seeking a solution to the question of sustainable domestic financing for the HIV response by integrating it into existing national health systems, as external HIV funders prepare to withdraw in an era of competing priorities both at home and in development terms, and the strained fiscal environment.

Normatively, the case for UHC is unassailable, whether considered in terms of human rights, human decency, political responsibility, international and global security or as a means to the fulfilment of the non-health requisites of sustainability.[16] Many countries have embraced UHC, and the World Health Organization and World Bank have provided technical assistance on UHC to more than 100 countries since 2010. While UHC is a matter of concern for countries of all sizes, down to the smallest island states, it is worth noting that the BRICS (Brazil, Russian India, China and South Africa) countries, representing around half of the global population, are all engaged in health system reforms designed to extend, deepen or otherwise improve health service coverage for their populations, while simultaneously working on ways to increase financial protection for those availing themselves of health services.

As a target of the SDGs, UHC has much to offer. First, it provides a platform for a more integrated organization of states' health sector. The broad set of 13 SDG targets for health, as well as health elements in many other targets, are broad, but the UHC rationale is that there should not be a continuance of the fragmented silo approaches that characterized much of the health MDGs. Second, the SDGs and UHC are intrinsically about improving equity; as such, using UHC as a common strategic framework monitoring platform ensures a continuous focus on health equity. Third, the health goal is closely linked to many of the other social, economic and environmental SDGs. Inter-sectoral action, including a major emphasis on promotion and prevention within health responses, is urgently needed. To end poverty and boost shared prosperity, countries need robust, inclusive economic growth. To drive growth, they need to build human capital through investments in health, education and social protection for all their citizens.

However, the road to UHC is by no means smooth, and in most of the countries newly embracing a UHC agenda, commitment to the general idea is balanced by at least as much concern regarding how exactly to move forward. The principles expressed in the WHO definition of UHC are a vitally important ideal and a helpful organizing principle, but there is not yet a widely agreed understanding of what the particulars of coverage and care must comprise in order for any nation's health system to count as 'universal'[17]—no standard system performance or health outcome measures for an adequately functioning UHC. Consequently, the term 'universal health coverage' can accommodate a very wide range in terms of: the extent, quality and accessibility of services; the medical conditions and/or financial status which in some cases trigger entitlement; the socio-cultural and socio-economic factors which shape accessibility and use[18]; and the means by which UHC is financed, including the following: national systems supported by general or targeted taxation; partially state-subsidized systems, but with user fees at the point of use, or for some services; health insurance schemes which might entail general or case-specific public support; and private systems which have some degree of mandated, public responsibilities.

As a step towards narrowing the concept, in December 2014 the WHO outlined in general terms its understanding of the conditions to be met for a community or country to achieve universal health coverage[19]:

1. A strong, efficient, well-run health system that meets priority health needs through people-centred integrated care (including services for HIV, tuberculosis, malaria, non-communicable diseases, maternal and child health) by:

   - informing and encouraging people to stay healthy and prevent illness;

- detecting health conditions early;
- having the capacity to treat disease; and
- helping patients with rehabilitation.

2. Affordability: a system for financing health services so people do not suffer financial hardship when using them. This can be achieved in a variety of ways.
3. Access to essential medicines and technologies to diagnose and treat medical problems.
4. A sufficient capacity of well-trained, motivated health workers to provide the services to meet patients' needs based on the best available evidence.

Whatever the specifics of each country's approach to UHC, the familiar difficulties which beset all UHC systems are (or would be) amplified for low-income countries: the unresolvable tensions between extent of coverage and costs; the fact that the means of securing and maintaining adequate levels of funding must be politically sanctioned as much as medically determined; and the very considerable challenges of simultaneously universalizing and strengthening health systems which are so often weak, patchy, and poorly managed, administered and monitored.[20] In addition, health systems in lower-income countries, regardless of the degree to which they approach universality, face relatively high disease burdens exacerbated and sustained by poverty. This gives them considerably less adaptability for dealing with health emergencies (such as the 2015 Ebola outbreak) or for scaling up provision for any particular disease or condition. Moreover, in practice, there is nothing in the establishment of a country UHC system which in itself will prevent gaps and deficiencies opening up in one or both of comprehensiveness of coverage or the quality of care—a condition as evident in the more developed Organisation for Economic Co-operation and Development (OECD) countries (nearly all of which have universal or near-universal health coverage),[21] as in developing countries.

Universal Health Coverage and the HIV Response

For the WHO, a 'strong, efficient, well-run health system' is at the heart of universal health coverage. The need for health system strengthening was sharply emphasized most recently by the Ebola outbreak in West Africa, the severity of the outbreak being in large part due to weak health systems, including a lack of capacity in surveillance and response. As a result of that outbreak, basic health services such as vaccinations, maternal and child health services, and treatment for common conditions suffered and need to be restored, but longer-term, key health reforms must be implemented, including strengthening community systems and their linkages to district health services, with a view to providing promotion, prevention, treatment, rehabilitation and palliation without causing financial hardship. In other words, what is needed is universal health coverage, which not only implies basic quality health service and financial protection for all, but provides a foundation for resilient health systems that can quickly identify, respond to and recover from outbreaks and disasters, as well as address endemic and long-term health challenges.

Undoubtedly, the HIV response would benefit from stronger health systems. Basic SRH services such as family planning and maternal and child health services have, over decades, developed solid infrastructures in sub-Saharan Africa; in some cases this has made the conception and execution of integrated HIV/AIDS services feasible. Recent work examining the impact of Performance Based Financing for Health in Rwanda and additional investment in the health system to strengthen basic health services noted a positive contribution of these schemes to rapid scale-up of HIV services.[22] Similarly, there are numerous examples of how fragmented and weak health systems have made the implementation of HIV programmes slow or extremely difficult, despite the availability of abundant financial resources for HIV. Such problems are not confined to ART scale-up. Health systems failures are seen as being at the root of the disappointing outcomes of tuberculosis (TB) control strategies (Directly Observed Treatment, Short-Course, or DOTS), Integrated Management of Childhood Illness (IMCI) and the integration of reproductive health services.[23] To attempt to address this, health funding in some areas has moved from disease-specific programming towards a Sector Wide Approach (SWA), an approach explored even by a highly disease-specific funding agency, the Global Fund for AIDS, TB and Malaria.[24]

Issues and Challenges

Notwithstanding the above, the Joint United Nations Programme on HIV and AIDS (UNAIDS) Fast Track agenda to ending AIDS as a public health concern by 2030 was not predicated on the integration of AIDS financing, management or organization/service delivery with national health systems, or, by extension, was it predicated on health systems strengthening. Whilst acknowledging the challenges that weak health systems can pose to progressing aspects of the HIV response (as mentioned above), the notable success in extending antiretroviral treatment (ART) coverage over the past decade has been achieved largely in the absence of strong health systems. Indeed, the UNAIDS Fast Track agenda to meet the goal of ending AIDS was instead based on rapidly and intensively upscaling its vertical HIV testing and treatment delivery systems to achieve 90 per cent of people living with HIV knowing their HIV status, 90 per cent of people who know their status receiving treatment and 90 per cent of people on HIV treatment having a suppressed viral load so their immune system remains strong and they are no longer or much less infectious—in 2020. The outcomes are set to fall well short of those targets.[25]

The argument for vertical programming persists because, in most low- and lower-middle-income countries, national health systems remain far too weak to deliver an effective HIV response, much less the planned increase in intensity of HIV programming over the next 15 years. But in the current climate, planning for a broad, international extension of UHC and health systems strengthening is not a viable proposition: 'For the 49 Low-Income Countries, it [was] estimated that between 2015 and 2019 there [would be] a $240 billion resource gap between [total health expenditure] and fiscal need for Universal Health Coverage (about 30 per cent of the total fiscal need), or a $550 billion resource gap if private expenditures on health [were] not included (about 70 per cent of the fiscal need).'[26] This, furthermore, raises a second issue of the feasibility of concurrently implementing health systems strengthening-based Universal Health Coverage (minus the HIV component) and the vertical response-based Fast Track to ending AIDS. The pressure on the financial, institutional and human resources of pursuing both agendas independently and simultaneously would most likely be to the detriment of one or other agenda, or both.

In addition to financial considerations, while most will agree the ideal is for the HIV response to be integrated into national health systems and other relevant sectoral services, many would caution against premature integration. A strong argument to support the continuation of vertical programming over the next 15 years is that it aims to move the HIV epidemic, and thereby the response, to a point where the response can be effectively integrated into the health system, that is, the point at which the epidemic is under control and AIDS is no longer a public health concern.

While health systems strengthening is at the heart of universal health coverage, presently, UHC remains at a largely conceptual stage in low- and lower-middle-income countries—an 'aspirational goal'—and it may take years before a version of UHC reaches implementation stage at the country level.

Even if countries were able to fund UHC and expedite the process from concept to implementation plan, the human resources required to deliver a stronger health system would take significant time to develop. The long lead time in training many categories of health professional—a lead time that is, in part, dictated by the pace of human ability to obtain and practice knowledge and skills—means that even well-planned, well-funded programmes of teaching and training would result in a relatively slow expansion of skilled domestic human resources for health.[27] The ambitious 90-90-90 Fast Track targets are extremely resource-intensive, particularly in the initial years of the Fast Track timeframe; UNAIDS acknowledges that 'to fast-track national [HIV] responses, extensive mobilization of human, institutional and financial resources will be needed.'[28] Possible outcomes of an integrated HIV/essential health services approach for human resources for health include the HIV response competing with other priority health services for limited human resources, and being left short; or perhaps more likely, the machinery that has built up around the HIV response over the past 15 years will dominate the implementation of any UHC agenda and appropriate a disproportionate share of human resources, to the detriment of other essential health services.

Even so, the human resources for HIV under a UHC approach would further diminish progress on the Fast Track agenda, which has struggled from the start. This is because an inevitably cumbersome national health system lacks the agility and responsiveness of a vertical programme. Essentially, by the time health systems in low- and lower-middle-income countries have the capacity to deliver the necessary level of response to 'end AIDS,' the critical window of opportunity we have before us since 2015 to act against AIDS may well have passed us by. UNAIDS projects the cost of inaction over the 2015–20 period will be huge: the lost opportunity to save 21 million lives, and prevent an additional 28 million people living with HIV by 2030, at an additional cost of US$24 billion every year for antiretroviral therapy.[29] The imperative to 'act now' in intensifying the AIDS response, before the challenge becomes so great we have little hope of containing it in the foreseeable future, means effectively that Fast Track cannot conceivably be delivered under a UHC integrated health systems agenda, even in the years after 2020.

This then invites the question of what kind of HIV response might be envisaged under UHC? Where the HIV response has been delivered in any meaningful way through vertical programming for at least the past decade, if not longer, the ministries of finance have little to no experience of financing the response, and the ministries of health have focused their efforts on other health concerns. A Minister of Finance of a high HIV prevalence African country explained the implications of moving from a United States President's Emergency Plan for AIDS Relief (PEPFAR)-funded vertical programme, to largely domestic financing of the HIV response:

> I am aware of PEPFAR and the importance of this programme for us, of course, as are all my colleagues in government, but as Minister of Finance I cannot tell you with any certainty how much, to whom and with what effect PEPFAR funds have been implemented in my country. At one level, it is a success of the AIDS response that it is able to function so effectively outside of government, but, in consequence, any changes involving greater country ownership will necessitate long-term government planning and this takes time. I cannot see how we can make such changes quickly, while sustaining and increasing the effectiveness and efficiency of the AIDS response.[30]

While low- and lower-middle-income countries may look to efficiency savings, borrowing, or additional income generation to close the projected total health expenditure resource gaps noted earlier, they are highly unlikely to succeed in funding the ideal UHC package, leading to inevitable prioritization. Without international disease-specific funding for HIV and a dedicated machinery to ensure and service the priority status of the HIV response, there is considerable risk that the HIV response will not be prioritized as the largest and most pressing SRH issue in sub-Saharan Africa, especially in countries with epidemics that are concentrated in key populations—notably sex workers, injecting drug users, men who have sex with men and prisoners. While politicians may possibly be aware of the longer-term implications of failing to address the epidemic in these key populations, notably the risk of a concentrated epidemic becoming generalized, their four-to-five-year elected terms are not conducive to prioritizing politically contentious, and largely 'hidden,' population groups over the larger citizenry.

Even in countries with generalized epidemics, the success of antiretro-viral drugs (ARVs) in keeping people living with HIV (PLHIV) healthy in many high-prevalence countries, coupled with the persistent stigma of HIV which often results in non-disclosure of HIV status, means the HIV epidemic is now much less visible for people in real terms. In a sense, ARVs are masking the scale of the problem, and weakening the rationale for the intensification of the AIDS response over the next 5–15 years: the fact that the number of new HIV infections exceeds the number of people being enrolled on antiretroviral therapy (ART)[31] and that challenges in ART adherence mean a rise in drug-resistant HIV and the need for much more expensive (i.e., unaffordable) second- and third-line ARV treatments at the inevitable expense of other basic health concerns, will likely have little purchase amongst an electorate that is, in large part, living day to day. As such, while the medical and human rights impetus for establishing UHC in low- and lower-middle-income countries cannot reasonably be contested, it is important that the enterprise should not be regarded as a quick means of lessening donor dependency for the fight against HIV and AIDS.

Reconciling UHC-Driven Integration and Dedicated HIV/ AIDS Responses

The relationship between HIV and AIDS services and country health systems is by no means dichotomous; in fact, there are efficiency gains to be had by more effectively coordinating overlapping services (treatment of TB and hepatitis C; screening; laboratory testing; the distribution of medicines).[32] Conditions certainly support this: a case study analysing the shift to second-line drugs in South Africa as treatment programmes mature suggested that 94 per cent of the costs per patient will likely be attributable to drugs, laboratory testing, and clinic and pharmacy services.[33] It remains the case that the kinds of scale-up at the heart of the 2030 'end AIDS' strategy will require a great deal of health systems strengthening in many of the most important affected areas/communities, both in clinical and supporting medical functions. However, although this might suggest that a strategically directed, more horizontal approach to HIV/AIDS funding is appropriate, the extent and continuing progress of the disease and the necessarily expansive nature of the 2030 strategy mean that the response will need to remain essentially vertical, at least for the worst-affected countries.

This notwithstanding, there are no easy options in deliberating between vertical versus horizontal approaches in the years to come. As the earlier quoted passage from an African Finance Minister points out, the largest part of donor financing in his country, PEPFAR, was conducted as an externally generated and directed extra-governmental initiative, not as a partnership. The prospect of a dramatic reduction in funding, combined with this and other recipient governments' limited and essentially parallel engagement with AIDS could scarcely be worse preparation for 'country ownership' and integration of the HIV response into SSA national health systems. It is clear that funding, on however large a scale, does not obviate the need for true partnerships and inclusive governance.

If the UNAIDS Fast Track agenda (or some adaptation of it) is to be prioritized over Universal Health Coverage, then, as far as possible, the AIDS response should actively seek to advance other priority health and development challenges identified under UHC and the SDGs. While some have argued that the unprecedented attention and vertical funding for HIV has undermined or slowed health systems strengthening, it should be remembered that in previous decades, the reality of weak and under-resourced health systems in most of the world and limited access to basic health services for the majority of the population were common phenomena before the HIV response. More importantly, there is evidence that, if managed correctly, the HIV response can be a unique opportunity to strengthen the wider health sector through integration of services and promoting primary health care. As Dr Margaret Chan, WHO Director-General until 2017 noted: 'I regard universal health coverage as the single most powerful concept that public health has to offer. It is inclusive. It unifies services and delivers them in a comprehensive and integrated way, based on primary health care.'[34] Pilot studies and demonstration projects have been conducted on the integration of HIV and SRH services (family planning in particular) which hold some promise that under the right conditions and with careful planning, integration and health systems strengthening can be advanced in tandem.[35]

And there is evidence that a public health approach to delivering HIV treatment has had a positive impact on the availability of primary health-care services in general. For example, in Rwanda, during the past decade, the platforms designed to scale up HIV interventions have been used to strengthen primary care and to expand a growing package of health services across the country in an equitable way.[36] Health facilities originally constructed with donor funding earmarked for the HIV response were tasked with integrated primary care, and national supply chains conceived to assist ART programmes were harnessed to deliver drugs and reagents for a wide range of conditions. Furthermore, in Botswana, cervical cancer is one of the leading causes of premature death among women, particularly those who are HIV-positive. Limited cytology laboratory screening capacity for cervical cancer meant patients were being diagnosed late, with advanced or terminal stage disease. In 2013, the Government of Botswana introduced into HIV clinics lower-cost, but equally effective, 'see and treat' screening procedures, along with cryotherapy to destroy abnormal tissue in the cervix by freezing it. Moreover, since the high incidence of cervical cancer in Botswana is linked to a sexually transmitted infection caused by the human papillomavirus, the targeted use of HIV prevention interventions, such as promotion of use of condoms, avoiding harmful use of alcohol and male circumcision, are also likely to help prevent cervical cancer, along with HPV vaccination for school-age girls.

African Regionalism and SRH

The history of African regionalism is a complex one—at the thematic level, involving the post-independence re-configuration of states, economic development and human security; and as with most other forms of regionalism, the African varieties exhibit enduring tensions between state interests and sensitivities about sovereignty against the hoped-for benefits of collective and integrative action. Moreover, the all-inclusive, continental African Union notwithstanding,

> regionalization in Africa has not been singular and its institutional expression is not monolithic. The rise in number and centrality of sub-regional political communities across Africa emphasises the importance of disaggregating the notion of region in the African context. Whilst continental projects capture a broad conception of region, the identities associated to sub-regional bodies are strong and their relevance to underwriting human protection has been vital.[37]

This variety of regionalisms presents distinct advantages as well as challenges when dealing with the enactment of norms agreed at a global level,[38] and while the largest portion of African regional initiatives have been devoted to economic development cooperation and to forms of national security, they also exhibit consistent accord with the principal tenets of universal human rights, out of which both the SDGs and the MDGs arose. At the same time, no African regional organization has any supranational authority; and disparities in size, wealth and power even within regional groupings do not always manifest in terms of hegemonic authority or socially progressive regional agendas.

Sub-Saharan regions carry a range of uniquely difficult combinations of infectious disease burdens (HIV/AIDS not least), poverty and a range of structural impediments to enacting SRH. The Southern African Development Community (SADC) is the largest and best-established sub-regional intergovernmental organization in the region, but successive organizational changes and its primary focus on economic growth and regional integration have placed health as a logical rather than immediately pressing, programmatic requirement for economic development. However, SADC has produced policy documents on health, from the 1999 SADC Protocol on Health to its Sexual and Reproductive Health Business Plan for the SADC Region 2011–2015.[39] The intended outcome of the latter was in line with SADC's integrative ethos: to 'deliver harmonized, comprehensive, sustainably resourced and evidence-informed SRH policies, programs and services in response to agreed regional and global SRH commitments and targets.' Subsequently, SADC adopted an integrated business plan for HIV, SRH, TB and Malaria 2016–20 with a budget of US$45 million. However, no funding was secured for the implementation of the plan and the 2017 Regional Budget Summit 'highlighted resource challenges, low levels of capacity, poor planning and coordination across various levels, and in some cases limited political will, which undermine the ability and confidence of government officials and parliamentarians to adequately perform their roles effectively and timeously.'[40]

But from this faltering start, in 2018 SADC produced the SRHR Strategy for the SADC Region (2019–2030) which has as its vision, '[To] ensure that all people in the SADC region enjoy a healthy sexual and reproductive life, have sustainable access, coverage and quality SRHR services, information and education, and are fully able to realize and exercise their SRH rights, as an integral component of sustainable human development in the SADC region.'[41] This is discussed further below.

The African Union is similarly disposed, but it has uniquely inclusive continental standing. Following the African Union Continental Policy Framework on Sexual and Reproductive Health and Rights (2005), the Maputo Plan of Action (2006)[42] was published, which had as its 'expected outcome' 'provid[ing] a framework from which countries can draw inspiration. This will not require the elaboration of new strategies but simply the incorporation of elements of this strategy into the existing ones.' The Maputo Action Plan was costed at US$16 billion for three years, a figure the report says is 'indicative of the scale of the required effort and should mobilize an appropriate response by governments, donors, civil society and the private sector.' While the plan was elaborated and highly relevant, but with the financial burden and urgency of health issues throughout much of SSA—and now, the still larger financial demands of the SDGs— there was little prospect that the required funds would be forthcoming from member states' budgets.

Similarly, the East African Health Research Commission (EAHRC), established in 2008, is a formal institution of the East African Community (EAC), with 'the mission to coordinate, conduct, and promote the conduct of health research in the region, and source, gather and disseminate findings from research for policy formulation and practice.'[43] It might be tempting to suppose that African regional organizations' commitments to SRH are at worst exercises in normative conformity; and at best, sincere but lacking the bureaucratic strength, political authority and practical resources to convert pledges and aspirations into programmes. However, although there is a great deal more to actionable normative consensus than formal governmental and organizational ascent, it is easy to overlook the worth and importance of the work Africa's regional organizations must conduct not only to secure coherence within and between themselves, but also to mediate the tensions between global/international positions and African sensitivities and aspirations.

The AU's African Peer Review Mechanism (APRM)[44] leads in this work, described by one analyst as follows: 'The APRM is an uneasy and unstable compromise, indicating a highly ambivalent relationship between African and global international societies. This relationship has to be understood in the context of an unequal global international society, dominated by a number of core states with an increasingly solidarist governance agenda, as well as the attempts of a largely pluralist African international society to manage its demands.'[45] The APRM does not deal directly with SRHR under any of its current four thematic areas, but it is implicit in the AU's visionary and ambitious Agenda 2063[46]; and the work it conducts on harmonizing standards of governance and forwarding its own forms of normative expectation are an essential prelude to the realization of the global goals—SRHR included—to which the AU's member states are formally committed.

CONCLUSION: COMPLEX ISSUES, LARGE COMMITMENTS, INCREMENTAL PROGRESS

Normative alignment around the main tenets of sexual and reproductive health is a significant advance.

The African Union's own commitments to sexual and reproductive health are the best measure of the extent to which the gradual growth and expression of an international consensus has been internalized. Indeed, the understanding that large improvements in SRH are integral to development has not merely been acknowledged, but asserted—a point about which the SRHR Strategy for the SADC Region (2019–2030) is explicit. Similarly, the developmental aspects of comprehensive SRH are also at the heart of the African Union Roadmap on Harnessing the Demographic Dividend through Investments in Youth.[47]

The disappointments of unrealized strategic-level declarations and the reluctance of SSA states to acknowledge health as a human right are not fixed impediments to further progress in SRH, any more than they are for the larger human rights regime. Beneath the highly visible failures of attempts to enact policy on unconsolidated normative ground are the countless ways in which progressive norms grow to become lived expectation for individuals and communities—what one study has termed their 'socialization'—'the process through which principled ideas become norms, which in turn influence the behaviour and domestic structure of states.'[48] For a matter as large as the advancement of sexual and reproductive health in sub-Saharan Africa, progress will always be uneven, at times discontinuous and subject to a variety of unsupportive conditions, ranging from the continued scourge of HIV to funding shortfalls. One important indicator of the ways that states' formal commitments can be pressed to enactment is through the courts, now a familiar recourse, including SSA states.[49]

Another promising initiative which is part of the SADC SRHR Strategy is its production of a 'scorecard' to monitor progress[50]—evidently a determination to enact as much of the Agenda as possible. In its detail, the scorecard is an advance over the MDG targets. Its list of indicators comprises: indicator; definition; rationale; alignment with strategic outcome and target; frequency of reporting; and data sources. Moreover, ten outcomes, each aligned with a specific SDG goal, are to be fast tracked. It cannot be realistically expected that as SDG 3.3 also specifies, HIV and AIDS will be ended as a public health threat by 2030, yet the aspiration and routinely monitored progress towards that goal are essential for the entire SRH enterprise.

The concept of health as a human right together with health rights as citizen entitlements have begun to feature in recent strategic-level documents—the former albeit without elaboration. This is not necessarily either evasive or regressive, as governments seek to advance various forms of SRH allowance and provision without provoking a backlash. Rights and the language of rights can sometimes require a form of strategic framing, concentrating on specific issues rather than encompassing rights language which can appear open-ended and threatening to established cultural norms. Rights and the broader meanings of rights are sometimes ushered in unbidden, as part of a general alignment with norms and practices. Of course, it still matters that the human right to health continues to receive its due advocacy. Currently, the realms of health rights and policy-making are intermittently interactive rather than congruent.

HIV is inescapably at the heart of sexual and reproductive health in sub-Saharan Africa and will continue to shape how other health priorities (including SRH) are accommodated, how health systems are configured and how they are funded.

It is notable that the African Union Roadmap on Harnessing the Demographic Dividend through Investments in Youth[51] omits any mention of HIV and AIDS bar a reference to the commitment in *Africa 2063*: 'Agenda 2063 "commits member states to integrate sexual and reproductive health and rights, family planning and HIV/AIDS services through reinforcing action on earlier commitments to enhance maternal, newborn and child health status, ensuring the integration necessary to facilitate synergies between HIV/AIDS, TB, Malaria and Maternal, Newborn and Child Health programmes."' Its own 'key actions and deliverables' are a full and admirably direct SRH agenda—but even within the context of 'Investing in Youth,' the absence of the unavoidable impact of the continuing struggle against HIV and AIDS is surprising:

- Establish and promote integrated adolescent and youth friendly health services in public and private health facilities, school clinics and other venues, with adequate services for sexual and reproductive health.

- Prioritize national investments to ensure universal access to family planning services, including expanding the use of modern contraceptives as stated in the Extended Maputo Plan of Action on Sexual and Reproductive Health and Rights (2016–2030) and reiterated by Article 14(g) of the Maputo Protocol on the Rights of Women.
- Foster sustainable investments in health systems, including in human resources and infrastructure, with the goal of enhancing access to quality health services for all and guaranteeing adequate financing for the health sector in line with the Abuja commitments and address morbidities that undermine quality of life and productivity of the workforce.
- Scale up the promotion and implementation of policies, community engagement strategies and behavioural change measures to enhance the reproductive rights of women and adolescent girls and their access to sexual and reproductive health education, information and services.
- Promote policies and programmes to improve child survival, for example, increasing immunization coverage, integrated management of childhood illness (IMCI) and improving child nutrition among others.
- Scale up age-appropriate and culturally sensitive comprehensive education on sexual and reproductive health in order to avert many complications and challenges associated with unintended pregnancies, sexually transmitted infections and its consequent impact on the development and well-being of young people, for in and out of school youth and implement innovative behavioural change programmes using new media and technology.
- Foster inter-sectoral action for health at all levels (state and non-state) in a manner that demonstrates broad stewardship towards all actions conducive and necessary for improvement in reproductive, maternal, newborn, child and adolescent health.
- Create an enabling environment by empowering communities and strengthening the role of men in improving access to sexual reproductive health and reproductive rights services.

'Foster[ing] sustainable investments in health systems with the goal of enhancing access to quality health services for all' cannot realistically be abstracted from the full costs of HIV and AIDS, not least because the necessary funding is not adequate even now; because HIV high-prevalence states are very dependent on insecure donor assistance; and because, as we have seen, the impetus towards universal health coverage and the hoped-for cost savings that would come from integrating HIV/AIDS services into national health systems are up against the continuing severity of the pandemic and the weaknesses of existing SSA health systems.

Advances in key SRH indicators in SSA have continued throughout the course of the AIDS pandemic—and highlighting the non-AIDS SRH agenda remains important, especially all aspects of advancing gender equality; however, the kinds of SRH agendas that have now become common currency both globally and within SSA will need to grapple with and reconcile HIV and AIDS initiatives against other SRH priorities. They are largely complementary, but the impacts of non-AIDS SRH programmes are likely to be gradual, at a time when we have still not brought the rate of new HIV infections under control.

Biomedical initiatives and interventions for SRH are necessary, but not sufficient for what are essentially issues of human relatedness.

No one could sensibly dispute the scale of the achievement and the worth of some 20 million lives saved because of antiretroviral treatments for HIV positive people, the reduction in mother-to-child transmission of AIDS, or the medical services involved in the full range of SRH debilities. But the wellsprings of sexual and reproductive ill health are in unequal gender relations, risky behaviours, discriminatory practices which cause the most vulnerable to avoid health services, and adolescents uncertain about sexuality and safe sex—in other words, in the values, perceptions and complex interactions of individuals.

But there is a strong counter-current that emphasizes approaches that seek 'solutions' that are both direct and quantifiable. But AIDS and other STDs are manifestations of human conditions and interactions; human affairs are messy and human perceptions and motivations are often opaque. Without disputing the importance of scientific and biomedical strategies for dealing with AIDS and other STDs, sexual and reproductive health in the largest senses cannot be treated with a 'silver bullet.' The further difficulty with approaches that seek to 'fix' issues is that the underlying ideology has broader ramifications:

Contrary to broader conceptualisations of HSS [health systems strengthening] that emphasise social and political dimensions, GAVI's [the global

Vaccine Alliance] HSS support has become emblematic of the so-called 'Gates approach' to global health, focused on targeted technical solutions with clear, measurable outcomes. In spite of adopting rhetoric supportive of 'holistic' health systems, [global health initiatives] like GAVI have come to capture the global debate about HSS in favour of their disease-specific approach and ethos.[52]

There is no need to have social and behavioural science studies and analyses freestanding from biomedical and scientific ones, and although it is not novel, the practice of combining them is still relatively uncommon.[53] There is much to be gained: as we saw, the efficacy of some forms of birth control is not sufficient to overcome some women's fears about their side effects; and overcoming resistance to voluntary male circumcision for HIV prevention does not require a stronger medical rationale, but an under-standing of cultural norms and individuals' perceptions. The social and behavioural sciences are not a useful complement to science and medicine, but integral to research and into proposed interventions about how sexual and reproductive health can be advanced most effectively. We cannot improve human lives without understanding how people live.

'Top-down' strategic initiatives are vitally important, but so too is the engagement, innovation and sustainability achievable in local and commu-nity levels.

It is in the values, beliefs and judgements of individuals that the very largest part of SRH vulnerabilities begin—in the relationships we contract that they find expression or are diminished, and at community levels that individual freedom and social order are reconciled. International and global proclamations do not create demand for SRH services or address the ways by which deleterious conditions, new laws, changing social norms and alternative ways of life can be absorbed or mediated. Without family and community ascent, children and adolescents cannot learn about sexu-ality and sexual relationships, or about their rights to health. It is by the slow change in the tenor of everyday interactions that sexual violence and sexual exploitation in its many varieties gradually become anathema or the stigma attached to unmarried women seeking contraception, family plan-ning, STD screening or abortion advice can be diminished. How else can our country-level plans be enacted except through both acceptance and engagement of those whom we hope to assist?

These points are widely accepted, if unevenly enacted programmati-cally, but they are likely to gain increased attention as the

SRH-UHC-AIDS crunch intensifies and hard choices at the political and funding levels begin to bite.[54]

And community-level advocates are the most heavily invested in partnerships, and for informing decisions about whether pilot programmes should be taken to scale through local knowledge and trust vital to evaluation projects.

Few things are more morally odious than the persistence of preventable suffering—with sexual and reproductive ill health perhaps only second to poverty, but to which it has obvious causal linkages. We cannot alter the deepest human propensities or perfect human societies but we can inform values, make knowledge freely available, act to bring gender equality to all aspects of social life, extend the reach and quality of our sexual and reproductive health services, drastically reduce mother and child mortality, and protect adolescents and young people from the worst vulnerabilities. That is the call of sexual and reproductive health rights, and sub-Saharan African states have accepted the very difficult challenges entailed in proclaiming their commitment to them. It is a considerable achievement in itself, which even partial successes in the years to come will validate.

NOTES

1. United Nations Economic and Social Council, 'Progress toward the Sustainable Development Goals, Report of the Secretary-General' (8 May 2019), E/2019/68, p. 11. Available at https://undocs.org/E/2019/68
2. Frances E. Baum, '"Never mind the logic, give me the numbers": Former Australian health ministers' perspectives on the social determinants of health,' *Social Science and Medicine* 87(2013), p.144.
3. An exception is Alan Davidson, *Social Determinants of Health: A Comparative Approach*, second Edition (Oxford: Oxford University Press, 2019). See also: Michael Marmot and Richard G. Wilkinson, *Social Determinants of Health*, Second Edition (Oxford: Oxford University Press, 2006); Adrian Bonner, *Social Determinants of Health* (Bristol: Policy Press, 2017). At the global/international levels, see: Audrey R. Chapman, *Global Health, Human Rights, and the Challenge of Neoliberal Policies* (Cambridge: Cambridge University Press, 2016), Chapter 5, 'Globalization, Health, and Human Rights,' pp. 153–99.
4. Mark Exworthy, 'Policy to tackle the social determinants of health: using conceptual models to understand the policy process,' *Health Policy and Planning* 23 (3) (2008), pp. 318–27. See also: Sanni Yaya, 'Socioeconomic Inequalities in the Risk Factors of Noncommunicable Diseases Among

Women of Reproductive Age in Sub-Saharan Africa: A Multi-Country Analysis of Survey Data,' *Public Health* (24 October 2018), available at: https://doi.org/10.3389/fpubh.2018.00307

5. Leen Vandecasteele, 'Life Course Risks or Cumulative Disadvantage? The Structuring Effect of Social Stratification Determinants and Life Course Events on Poverty Transitions in Europe,' *European Sociological Review* 27(2), April 2011, pp. 246–63; Rachel Stein Berman, Milani R. Patel, Peter F. Belamarich and Rachel S. Gross, 'Screening for Poverty and Poverty-Related Social Determinants of Health,' *Pediatrics in Review* 39(5) (May 2018), pp. 235–46.

6. World Bank, *Accelerating Poverty Reduction in Africa* (2019), pp. 1; 4. Available at: https://openknowledge.worldbank.org/handle/10986/32354

7. Ibid., p. 3. Italics original.

8. John W. McArthur and Krista Rasmussen, 'Change of pace: Accelerations and advances during the Millennium Development Goal era,' *World Development* 105 (2018), p. 142.

9. African Union, *Africa 2063*, Goals: https://au.int/en/agenda2063/goals

10. Ayesha B. M. Kharsany and Quarraisha A. Karim, 'HIV Infection and AIDS in Sub-Saharan Africa: Current Status, Challenges,' *Open AIDS* (10) (2016), p. 37.

11. WHO, *HIV, Universal Health Coverage and the Post-2015 Development Agenda* (WHO Department of HIV/AIDS), 2014.

12. El-Sadr WM, Abrams EJ. 'Scale-up of HIV care and treatment: can it transform healthcare services in resource-limited settings?', *AIDS* 2007, 21 Suppl 5:S65–70.

13. World Health Organization, http://www.who.int/health_financing/universal_coverage_definition/en/

14. United Nations Department of Economic and Social Affairs, Open Working Group proposal for Sustainable Development Goals, 2014, available at: https://sustainabledevelopment.un.org/focussdgs.html

15. WHO, What is Universal Health Coverage?, Q&A, December 2014. Accessed at: http://www.who.int/features/qa/universal_health_coverage/en/

16. UNGA resolution A/67/L.36; World Health Organization, World Health Report 2010: Health Systems Financing—The Path to Universal Coverage, available at: http://www.who.int/whr/2010/whr10_en.pdf?ua=1; see also The Commission on Macroeconomics and Health, Investing in Health for Economic Development (2001), available at: http://www.earth.columbia.edu/sitefiles/file/Sachs%20Writing/2002/GlobalHealthLink_2002_InvestinginHealthforEconDev_March2002.pdf; Elio Borgonovi and Amelia Compagni, 'Sustaining Universal Health

Coverage: The Interaction of Social, Political and Economic Sustainability,' *Value in Health* 16 (2013), S34–38, available at: http://www.valuein-healthjournal.com/article/S1098-3015(12)04157-5/pdf

17. However, the recently established Health for All Global Network (http://universalhealthcoverageday.org) lists the 'core tenets' of UHC as follows: Prioritize the poorest; increase reliance on public funding; reduce, if not eliminate out-of-pocket spending; and develop the health system. See also: Thomas O'Connell, Kumanan Rasanathan and Mickey Chopra, 'What does universal health coverage mean?' *The Lancet* 383 (2014), pp. 77–9.

18. In one Canadian study, 'On average, 40 per cent of people who died of HIV/AIDS-related causes during the study period had never accessed [ART] treatment. This finding is of particular concern, given that treatment is universal and provided free of charge in British Columbia.' Ruth Joy et al., 'Impact of Neighborhood-Level Socioeconomic Status on HIV Disease Progression in a Universal Health Care Setting,' *Journal of Acquired Immune Deficiency Syndromes*, 47(4), (1 April 2008), pp. 500–505.

19. WHO, What is Universal Health Coverage? Q&A, December 2014. Accessed at: http://www.who.int/features/qa/universal_health_coverage/en/

20. Dr Margaret Chan, Director-General of the World Health Organization, speech made to the Measurement and Accountability for Results in Health Summit, Washington, DC, 9 June 2015, available at: http://www.who.int/dg/speeches/2015/health-measurement-summit/en/

21. '[In OECD countries], unmet health care needs are still reported, most commonly among low-income groups.' Health at a Glance: OECD Indicators, 2013, Available at: http://www.oecd.org/els/health-systems/Health-at-a-Glance-2013-Chart-set.pdf

22. M. Schneidman and L. Rusa, 'Rwanda Performance Based Financing for Health,' Center for Global Development Working Group on Performance Based Incentives.

23. H. Schneider et al., 'Health systems and access to antiretroviral drugs for HIV in Southern Africa: service delivery and human resources challenges,' *Reproductive Health Matters* 14 (2006), pp. 12–23.

24. C. Dickinson et al., 'The Global Fund operating in a SWAp through a common fund: issues and lessons from Mozambique,' HLSP Institute (2007), available at: https://www.who.int/healthsystems/gf7.pdf

25. Jacob Levi et al., 'Can the UNAIDS 90-90-90 target be achieved? A systematic analysis of national HIV treatment cascades,' *BMJ Global Health* 1 (2016), Doi:10.1136/ bmjgh-2015-000010; Anneke Grobler et al., 'Progress of UNAIDS 90-90-90 targets in a district in KwaZuku natal, South Africa, with high HIV burden, in the HIPSS study: a household-based

complex multilevel community survey,' *The Lancet HIV* 4(11)(2017), pp. E505-E513.

26. Oxford Policy Management, 'Opportunities and challenges for the integration of health and HIV financing,' p. 4.

27. Di McIntyre and Filip Meheus, *Fiscal Space for Domestic Funding of Health and Other Social Services*, Paper 5, Centre on Global Health Security Working Group Papers, The Royal Institute of International Affairs, March 2014.

28. UNAIDS, Fast-Track: ending the AIDS epidemic by 2030, Geneva: UNAIDS, 2014, p. 19.

29. Ibid., p. 26.

30. Quote from interview with the Minister of Finance of an HIV high prevalence African country, conducted by author, 2 September 2015.

31. UNAIDS, 'AIDS at 30: Nations at a Crossroads' (2011), available at: http://reliefweb.int/sites/reliefweb.int/files/resources/aids-at-30.pdf

32. Dermot Mahler, 'Re-thinking global health sector efforts for HIV and tuberculosis epidemic control: promoting integration of programme activities within a strengthened health system,' *BMC Public health* 10:394 (2010), available at: http://www.biomedcentral.com/content/pdf/1471-2458-10-394.pdf

33. L. Long, M. Fox, I. Sanne and S. Rosen, 'The high cost of second-line antiretroviral therapy for HIV/AIDS in South Africa,' *AIDS* 24(6) (2010), pp. 915–19; see also: R. Hecht et al, 'Financing of HIV/AIDS programme scale-up in low-income and middle-income countries, 2009–31,' *The Lancet* 376 (9748) (2010), pp. 1254–60.

34. http://www.who.int/universal_health_coverage/en/

35. UNFPA and UNAIDS, 'Linking sexual and reproductive health and rights and HIV in Southern Africa: Demonstration projects in seven Southern African countries have scaled up effective models for strengthening integrated SRH and HIV policies, systems, and service delivery mechanisms' (2015), http://www.integrainitiative.org/wp/wp-content/ uploads/2015/10/Regional-booklet-final.pdf. 25 March 2017; see also the Special Issue of *Studies in Family Planning*, Research on integrating sexual and reproductive Health and HIV Services: Current Status, Future Challenges, Volume 48(2) (June 2017), pp. 89–219.

36. Sara Stulac et al., 'Capacity building for oncology programmes in sub-Saharan Africa: the Rwanda experience,' *The Lancet Oncology* 16(8), (August 2015), pp. e405–13.

37. Charles T. Hunt, 'African Regionalism & Human Protection Norms: An Overview,' *Global Responsibility to Protect* 8 (2016), p. 211.

38. C. Hartmann, 'Leverage and linkage: how regionalism shapes regime dynamics in Africa,' *Zeitschrift für Vergleichende Politikwissenschaft* (February 2016), Volume 10, Supplement 1, pp. 79–98.
39. SADC, Sexual and Reproductive Health Business Plan for the SADC Region 2011–2015. Available at: https://www.sadc.int/files/3613/5293/3504/SADC_Sexual_and_Reproductive_Health_Business_Plan_2011-2015.pdf
40. Regional Budget Summit on Strengthening Social Accountability in Health and Agriculture in Southern Africa (15 August 2017), available at: http://copsam.com/wp-content/uploads/2017/02/PSA-Annual-Budget-Summit-2017-Final-Report.pdf
41. The Sexual and Reproductive Health and Rights (SRHR) Strategy for the SADC Region, 2019–2030 (2018), available at: http://genderlinks.org.za/wp-content/uploads/2018/11/1-Final-signed-SADC-SRHR-Strategy-2019-2030.pdf
42. African Union Commission, Maputo Plan of Action for the Operationalisation of the Continental Policy Framework for Sexual and Reproductive Health and Rights, 2007–2010. (2006), available at: https://au.int/sites/default/files/newsevents/workingdocuments/27514-wd-mpoa_7-_revised_au_stc_inputs_may_se-rob-director_002.pdf
43. East African Community, http://www.eac.int/about/institutions/eahrc
44. African Peer Review Mechanism, available at: http://aprm-au.org
45. Elaine Shek Yan Tan, 'Interactions between African and Global International Societies: the African Peer Review Mechanism (APRM),' *Global Discourse* 5(3) (2015), p. 398; see also Yannis A. Stivachtis, 'Interrogating Regional International Societies: Questioning the Global International Society,' *Global Discourse* 5(3) (2015), pp. 327–40.
46. Agenda 63: The Africa We Want, http://www.un.org/en/africa/osaa/pdf/au/agenda2063.pdf
47. African Union Roadmap on Harnessing the Demographic Dividend through Investments in Youth, in response to AU Assembly Decision (Assembly/AU/Dec.601). Available at: https://addis.unfpa.org/sites/default/files/pub-pdf/AU%202017%20DD%20ROADMAP%20Final%20-%20EN_2.pdf
48. Thomas Risse and Kathryn Sikkink, 'The socialization of international human rights norms into domestic practices: introduction,' in Thomas Risse, Stephen C. Ropp and Kathryn Sikkink (eds), *The Power of Human Rights: International Norms and Domestic Change* (Cambridge: Cambridge University Press, 1999), p. 7.
49. Ebenezer Durojaye (ed), *Litigating the Right to Health in Africa: Challenges and Prospects* (Aldershot: Ashgate, 2015); Marius Pieterse, 'Health, Social Movements and Rights-based Litigation in South Africa,'

Journal of Law and Society 35(3) (2008), pp. 364–88. Note, however, that SRH litigation can cut both ways: María Angélica Peñas Defago and José Manuel Morán Faúndes, 'Conservative litigation against sexual and reproductive health policies in Argentina,' *Reproductive Health Matters* 22 (44) (2014), pp. 82–90.

50. SADC, Score Card for Sexual and Reproductive Health and Rights in the SADC Region: *Fast tracking the Strategy for SRHR in the SADC Region 2019–2030*, available at: https://genderlinks.org.za/wp-content/uploads/2018/11/SADC-SRHR-Final-Signed-Score-Card-221018.pdf

51. African Union Road Map, *op cit.*

52. Katerini T. Storeng, 'The GAVI Alliance and the "Gates approach" to health system strengthening,' *Global Public Health* 9(8) (2014), p. 865.

53. Amy Corneli et al., 'How Biomedical HIV Prevention Trials Incorporate Behavioral and Social Sciences Research: A Typology of Approaches,' *AIDS and Behavior* 23(2), (2019), pp. 2146–54; Carol S. Camlin and Janet Seeley, 'Qualitative research on community experiences in large HIV research trials: what have we learned?' *Journal of the International AIDS Society* 21(S7), (2018), pp. 55–9.

54. Deborah Jones, Stephen Weiss and Ndashi Chitalu, 'HIV Prevention in Resource Limited Settings: A Case Study of Challenges and Opportunities for Implementation,' *International Journal of Behavioral Medicine* 22 (2015), pp. 284–92; Donna M. Denno, 'Effective Strategies to Provide Adolescent Sexual and *Reproductive Health Services and to Increase Demand and Community Support,*' *Journal of Adolescent Health* 56 (2015) S22–S41.

Index[1]

[1] Note: Page numbers followed by 'n' refer to notes.

© The Author(s), under exclusive license to Springer Nature Singapore Pte Ltd. 2020
N. K. Poku, *Sexual and Reproductive Health and Rights in Sub-Saharan Africa*, Global Research in Gender, Sexuality and Health, https://doi.org/10.1007/978-981-15-8502-9